Transfusion in the Intensive Care Unit

Nicole P. Juffermans • Timothy S. Walsh
Editors

Transfusion
in the Intensive Care Unit

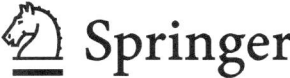 Springer

Editors
Nicole P. Juffermans
Department of Intensive Care L.E.I.C.A.
Academic Medical Center
Amsterdam
The Netherlands

Timothy S. Walsh
MRC Centre for Inflammation Research
University of Edinburgh
The Queens Medical Research Institute
Edinburgh
UK

ISBN 978-3-319-08734-4   ISBN 978-3-319-08735-1   (eBook)
DOI 10.1007/978-3-319-08735-1
Springer Cham Heidelberg New York Dordrecht London

Library of Congress Control Number: 2014950910

Printed on acid-free paper

Springer is part of Springer Science+Business Media (www.springer.com)

Contents

1 **Introduction** 1
Nicole P. Juffermans and Timothy S. Walsh

2 **Causes of Anemia in Critically Ill Patients** 5
Daniela Ortega and Yasser Sakr

3 **Red Blood Cell Transfusion Trigger in Sepsis** 13
Jean-Louis Vincent

4 **Red Blood Cell Transfusion Trigger in Cardiac Disease** 25
Parasuram Krishnamoorthy, Debabrata Mukherjee,
and Saurav Chatterjee

5 **Red Blood Cell Transfusion Trigger in Cardiac Surgery** 35
Gavin J. Murphy, Nishith N. Patel, and Jonathan A.C. Sterne

6 **Red Blood Cell Transfusion Trigger in Brain Injury** 45
Shane W. English, Dean Fergusson, and Lauralyn McIntyre

7 **Red Blood Cell Transfusion in the Elderly** 59
Matthew T. Czaja and Jeffrey L. Carson

8 **ScvO₂ as an Alternative Transfusion Trigger** 71
Szilvia Kocsi, Krisztián Tánczos, and Zsolt Molnár

9 **Alternatives to Red Blood Cell Transfusion** 77
Howard L. Corwin and Lena M. Napolitano

10 **Blood-Sparing Strategies in the Intensive Care Unit** 93
Andrew Retter and Duncan Wyncoll

11 **Massive Transfusion in Trauma** 101
Daniel Frith and Karim Brohi

12 **Transfusion in Gastrointestinal Bleeding** 121
Vipul Jairath

13 **Platelet Transfusion Trigger in the Intensive Care Unit** 139
D. Garry, S. Mckechnie, and S.J. Stanworth

14 FFP Transfusion in Intensive Care Medicine 151
David Hall and Timothy S. Walsh

15 Transfusion-Related Acute Lung Injury 161
Alexander P.J. Vlaar and Nicole P. Juffermans

16 Transfusion-Associated Circulatory Overload 171
Leanne Clifford and Daryl J. Kor

Index 183

Introduction

1

Nicole P. Juffermans and Timothy S. Walsh

Critically ill patients are frequently transfused, with 40–50 % of patients receiving a red blood cell transfusion during their stay in the intensive care unit (ICU) [1].

Current red blood cell transfusion practice in the ICU has largely been shaped by a landmark trial published in 1999, which taught us that a restrictive transfusion trigger is well tolerated in the critically ill and of particular benefit in the young and less severely ill [2]. Following this trial, a restrictive trigger has been widely adopted [3–5]. Nevertheless, transfusion rates in the ICU remain high, rendering blood transfusion part of everyday practice in the ICU.

Red blood cell transfusion rates in the ICU are high because many patients suffer moderately to severe anemia. Anemia is a hallmark of critical illness, occurring in up to 90 % of patients. The cause of anemia is multifactorial, but the presence of inflammation is an important contributor. As anemia usually develops early in the course of critical illness, the term "anemia of inflammation" has become interchangeable with the term "anemia of chronic disease," which may better describe the critically ill patient population. Transfusion of fresh frozen plasma (FFP) is also common practice in the ICU, with estimates of 12–60 % of patients receiving plasma during their stay [6, 7]. Frequent transfusion of FFP is due to a large proportion of patients with a coagulopathy and/or patients who experience or are considered at risk for bleeding [7, 8]. The reported wide variation in the practice of FFP transfusion suggests clinical uncertainty about best practice [7–9].

N.P. Juffermans (✉)
Department of Intensive Care Medicine, Academic Medical Center,
Room G3-206, Meibergdreef 9, 1105 AZ Amsterdam, The Netherlands

Laboratory of Experimental Intensive Care and Anesthesiology (L.E.I.C.A.),
Academic Medical Center, Amsterdam, The Netherlands
e-mail: n.p.juffermans@amc.uva.nl

T.S. Walsh
Department of Anaesthetics, Critical Care and Pain Medicine,
Edinburgh University, Edinburgh, UK

© Springer International Publishing Switzerland 2015
N.P. Juffermans, T.S. Walsh (eds.), *Transfusion in the Intensive Care Unit*,
DOI 10.1007/978-3-319-08735-1_1

Similarly, thrombocytopenia is a prevalent, occurring in up to 30 %, triggering platelet transfusion in 10 % of patients [7]. Taken together, transfusion of blood products is one of the most common therapies in the ICU.

It is increasingly clear that an association between transfusion and adverse outcome exists, including the occurrence of lung injury, multiple organ failure, thromboembolic events, and nosocomial infections. These associations are not restricted to the critically ill patient population, but the relation between blood transfusion and adverse outcome seems most apparent in this group [10], suggesting that critically ill patients may have specific features which render them susceptible to possible detrimental effects of a blood transfusion. Thereby, ICU physicians are advised to be restrictive with transfusion [11, 12]. A challenge in understanding the optimum use of blood products in the critically ill is delineating whether this association is causative or simply a result of the residual confounding and bias by indication which influences observational studies.

The dark side of these efforts to adhere to a restrictive practice to mitigate adverse effects of blood transfusion may be under-transfusion, which may be particularly relevant to the correction of anemia with red blood cells. Multiple studies have shown an association between anemia and adverse outcome, in a wide variety of patients, including brain injury and myocardial infarction [11, 13–16]. Thereby, both anemia and transfusion are unwanted conditions, posing a challenge to the treating physician, who wonders what to do with a low hemoglobin level. Transfuse, not transfuse, or consider an alternative treatment?

These observations underline the need for a careful assessment of whether risks of transfusion outweigh the perceived benefit. In other words, can a particular patient tolerate anemia? Tolerance to anemia differs between different populations, depending on physiologic state, diagnosis, comorbidity, and cause of anemia. Although guidelines advise taking age and other physiologic variables into consideration in the decision to transfuse [11, 12], studies which have compared different triggers in different settings have been limited, and the overall evidence base is weak. Red cell transfusion, in particular, is still strongly influenced by the landmark "TRICC" trial and applied in a "one-size-fits-all" fashion. This despite changes to the red cell product in many countries (the introduction of leucodepletion), improvements in other aspects of critical care (which might change the "signal-to-noise" ratio associated with blood transfusion), and the fact that the original trial was underpowered and stopped early having reached only half of the intended sample size.

In the last decade, several clinical trials have studied red blood cell transfusion triggers in various ICU patient populations. Also, large and well-conducted trials have been performed in specific conditions which are frequently present in the critically ill, including myocardial infarction or gastrointestinal bleeding. These studies empower the physician to take a personalized approach towards transfusion of red blood cells and are discussed in this book.

Also for FFP, the horizon has lightened up with data on efficacy of FFP in traumatic bleeding, which suggest that in traumatic bleeding, FFP should be given earlier and in greater quantities. An important trial on platelet transfusion to prevent bleeding was also recently published, although from the hemoncology setting.

A handbook which summarizes results from these recent trials on transfusion triggers was lacking. Here, we present a practical handbook on transfusion triggers in the ICU, which can be used in everyday practice. Chapters are written by leading researchers in the field from all over the globe. This book aims to facilitate a more tailor-made approach in specific ICU patient populations. In the absence of large randomized trials in specific subpopulations, such an approach will help decrease under-transfusion as well as unnecessary over-transfusion, thereby increasing efficacy of the use of available blood. We hope this book will help clinicians make rational individualized decisions, avoiding a "one-size-fits-all" transfusion practice and promoting personalized therapy. This book also provides practical information on alternatives to red blood cell transfusion, as well as means to limit loss of blood by phlebotomy. The most common adverse events are also discussed, again with a practical focus on management at the bedside.

Optimal care for a patient always requires clinical judgment of the treating physician, because individual patients may not fall within a clear recommendation. Nevertheless, we hope this book may support physicians in their everyday care for the critically ill.

References

1. Vincent JL, Piagnerelli M. Transfusion in the intensive care unit. Crit Care Med. 2006;34(5 Suppl):S96–101.
2. Hebert PC, Wells G, Blajchman MA, Marshall J, Martin C, Pagliarello G, Tweeddale M, Schweitzer I, Yetisir E. A multicenter, randomized, controlled clinical trial of transfusion requirements in critical care. Transfusion Requirements in Critical Care Investigators, Canadian Critical Care Trials Group. N Engl J Med. 1999;340(6):409–17.
3. Corwin HL, Gettinger A, Pearl RG, Fink MP, Levy MM, Abraham E, MacIntyre NR, Shabot MM, Duh MS, Shapiro MJ. The CRIT Study: Anemia and blood transfusion in the critically ill – current clinical practice in the United States. Crit Care Med. 2004; 32(1):39–52.
4. Vincent JL, Sakr Y, Sprung C, Harboe S, Damas P. Are blood transfusions associated with greater mortality rates? Results of the Sepsis Occurrence in Acutely Ill Patients study. Anesthesiology. 2008;108(1):31–9.
5. Vlaar AP, in der Maur AL, Binnekade JM, Schultz MJ, Juffermans NP. Determinants of transfusion decisions in a mixed medical-surgical intensive care unit: a prospective cohort study. Blood Transfus. 2009;7(2):106–10.
6. Reiter N, Wesche N, Perner A. The majority of patients in septic shock are transfused with fresh-frozen plasma. Dan Med J. 2013;60(4):A4606.
7. Stanworth SJ, Walsh TS, Prescott RJ, Lee RJ, Watson DM, Wyncoll D. A national study of plasma use in critical care: clinical indications, dose and effect on prothrombin time. Crit Care. 2011;15(2):R108.
8. Vlaar AP, in der Maur AL, Binnekade JM, Schultz MJ, Juffermans NP. A survey of physicians' reasons to transfuse plasma and platelets in the critically ill: a prospective single-centre cohort study. Transfus Med. 2009;19(4):207–12.
9. Watson DM, Stanworth SJ, Wyncoll D, McAuley DF, Perkins GD, Young D, Biggin KJ, Walsh TS. A national clinical scenario-based survey of clinicians' attitudes towards fresh frozen plasma transfusion for critically ill patients. Transfus Med. 2011;21(2):124–9.
10. Marik PE, Corwin HL. Efficacy of red blood cell transfusion in the critically ill: a systematic review of the literature. Crit Care Med. 2008;36(9):2667–74.

11. Napolitano LM, Kurek S, Luchette FA, Corwin HL, Barie PS, Tisherman SA, Hebert PC, Anderson GL, Bard MR, Bromberg W, Chiu WC, Cipolle MD, Clancy KD, Diebel L, Hoff WS, Hughes KM, Munshi I, Nayduch D, Sandhu R, Yelon JA. Clinical practice guideline: red blood cell transfusion in adult trauma and critical care. Crit Care Med. 2009;37(12):3124–57.
12. Retter A, Wyncoll D, Pearse R, Carson D, McKechnie S, Stanworth S, Allard S, Thomas D, Walsh T. Guidelines on the management of anaemia and red cell transfusion in adult critically ill patients. Br J Haematol. 2013;160(4):445–64.
13. Chatterjee S, Wetterslev J, Sharma A, Lichstein E, Mukherjee D. Association of blood transfusion with increased mortality in myocardial infarction: a meta-analysis and diversity-adjusted study sequential analysis. JAMA Intern Med. 2013;173(2):132–9.
14. Oddo M, Levine JM, Kumar M, Iglesias K, Frangos S, Maloney-Wilensky E, Le Roux PD. Anemia and brain oxygen after severe traumatic brain injury. Intensive Care Med. 2012;38(9):1497–504.
15. Sekhon MS, McLean N, Henderson WR, Chittock DR, Griesdale DE. Association of hemoglobin concentration and mortality in critically ill patients with severe traumatic brain injury. Crit Care. 2012;16(4):R128.
16. Villanueva C, Colomo A, Bosch A, Concepcion M, Hernandez-Gea V, Aracil C, Graupera I, Poca M, Alvarez-Urturi C, Gordillo J, Guarner-Argente C, Santalo M, Muniz E, Guarner C. Transfusion strategies for acute upper gastrointestinal bleeding. N Engl J Med. 2013; 368(1):11–21.

Daniela Ortega and Yasser Sakr

Abstract

Anemia is a common occurrence in critically ill patients and is associated with considerable morbidity and worse outcomes. The prevalence of anemia among critically ill patients is influenced by factors that include patient case mix, illness severity, and preexisting comorbidity. Several factors may lead to anemia in critically ill patients and the etiology of anemia in individual patients is commonly multifactorial and may be related either to the underlying disease process or occur as a consequence of diagnostic or therapeutic interventions in the intensive care unit (ICU). Anemia of chronic disease is the most important form of anemia related to preexisting morbidity on admission to ICU. Blood loss considerably contributes to the development of anemia during the ICU stay. Other factors that may lead to anemia in critically ill patients include reduced red blood cell (RBC) production, abnormal RBC maturation, decreased RBC survival, or excessive RBC destruction. This chapter reviews the possible etiologic factors of anemia with a special emphasis on the underlying pathophysiology of these factors.

2.1 Introduction

Anemia is a common occurrence in critically ill patients and is associated with considerable morbidity and worse outcomes [1, 2]. The prevalence of anemia among critically ill patients is influenced by factors that include patient case mix, illness severity, and preexisting comorbidity [3]. A cohort study of 3,534 patients admitted

D. Ortega, MD • Y. Sakr, MD, PhD (✉)
Department of Anesthesiology and Intensive Care, Friedrich-Schiller-University Hospital,
Erlanger Allee 103, 07743 Jena, Germany
e-mail: yasser.sakr@med.uni-jena.de

© Springer International Publishing Switzerland 2015
N.P. Juffermans, T.S. Walsh (eds.), *Transfusion in the Intensive Care Unit*,
DOI 10.1007/978-3-319-08735-1_2

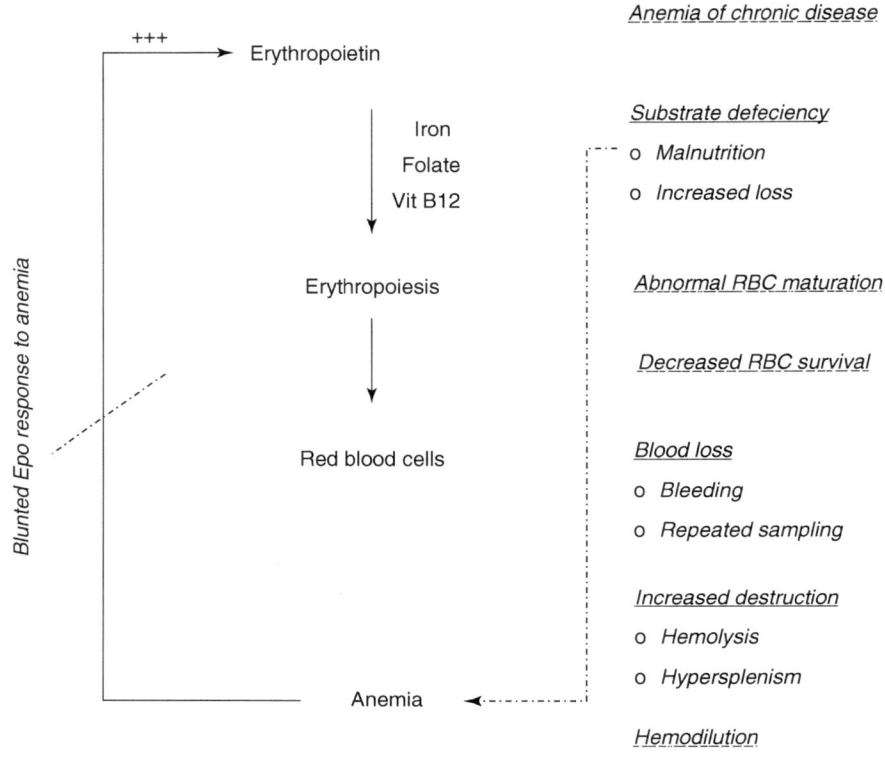

Fig. 2.1 Schematic diagram demonstrating the possible causes of anemia in critically ill patients

to Western European intensive care units (ICUs) reported that 63 % of patients had a hemoglobin concentration <12 g/dl at ICU admission and 29 % had hemoglobin concentrations <10 g/dl [1]. In this study, anemia was more frequent and severe in older patients. During the ICU stay, hemoglobin concentrations decreased on average by 0.66 g/dl/day for the first 3 days and by 0.12 g/dl/day thereafter. An early rapid decrease in hemoglobin values was also reported in a prospective observational single-center cohort study of patients present for more than 24 h in the ICU [4]. Another study found that 77.4 % of all ICU survivors were anemic (defined as hemoglobin concentration < 13 g/dl for men and < 11.5 g/dl for women) when discharged home from the hospital and 32.5 % had a hemoglobin concentration <10 g/dl. Fifty percent of patients who spent >7 days in the ICU had hemoglobin concentrations <10 g/dl at hospital discharge [5].

    Several factors contribute to anemia in critically ill patients (Fig. 2.1). The etiology of anemia in individual patients is commonly multifactorial [3] and may be related either to the underlying disease process or occur as a consequence of diagnostic or therapeutic interventions in the ICU. The most important factors are discussed in the following section.

2.2   Anemia of Chronic Disease

Anemia of chronic disease (ACD) is a common form of anemia that occurs in patients suffering from longstanding and/or advanced chronic disease [6]. Patients can be considered to have ACD when they present the following: (1) a chronic infection or inflammation, autoimmune disease or malignancy or renal disease; (2) a hemoglobin concentration <13 g/dl for men and <12 g/dl for women; and (3) a low transferrin saturation (<20 %), but normal or increased serum ferritin concentration (>100 ng/ml) or low serum ferritin concentration (30–100 ng/ml) [7]. Measurement of reticulocyte counts, endogenous erythropoietin (EPO) secretion (ratio of observed EPO to expected EPO), and serum creatinine (glomerular filtration) may be helpful in defining the cause of ACD. Because critically ill patients often have multiple comorbidities, this type of anemia may contribute to the prevalent low hemoglobin levels described on admission to the ICU in large epidemiologic studies [1, 2]. Fifty percent of patients admitted to ICUs with hemoglobin concentrations <10 g/dl have a history of either acute bleeding or ACD [1].

2.3   Blood Loss

Blood loss is a significant cause of anemia in intensive care patients. Potential sources of blood loss are diagnostic blood sampling and hemorrhage.

2.3.1   Phlebotomy Losses

Early studies found that, on average, a critically ill patient lost 1–2 units of blood through blood sampling during their hospital stay or up to 30 % of the total blood transfused in the ICU [8]. More recent data indicate that 30–40 ml are removed in blood samples per 24 h, with more blood sampled in sicker patients and those receiving renal replacement therapy [1]. Laboratory testing plays a critical role in diagnosis and guiding appropriate patient management during critical illness; a recent study in trauma patients suggested that laboratory testing is becoming more frequent with an increase in the number of blood tests ordered and blood volumes drawn in 2009 compared to 2004 [9].

2.3.2   Hemorrhagic Losses

There are many potential sources of bleeding in critically ill patients. Gastrointestinal bleeding may play a less important role than in the past with more widespread use of prophylaxis and rapid resuscitation and management, but some groups of patients, for example, those receiving mechanical ventilation or with coagulopathy and renal failure [10], remain at higher risk of bleeding. A recent study in Australia and New Zealand reported that bleeding was the reason for transfusion in 46 % of transfusion events [11].

2.4   Reduced Red Cell Production

Red blood cell (RBC) production, or erythropoiesis, occurs in the bone marrow and is controlled by EPO, a 165 amino acid glycoprotein hormone produced by interstitial fibroblasts in the kidney [12]. EPO promotes the proliferation and differentiation of early erythroid progenitors in the bone marrow into mature erythrocytes. Effective erythropoiesis requires various factors, including iron, zinc, folate and vitamin B_{12}, thyroxine, androgens, cortisol, and catecholamines [13]. RBC formation occurs at a basal rate of 15–20 ml/day under physiological conditions but can increase up to tenfold after hemolysis or heavy blood loss [14].

2.4.1   Substrate Deficiency

Iron deficiency may play a major role in decreased RBC production in critically ill patients. Around 70 % of the iron in the body is located within RBC hemoglobin. The body absorbs 1–2 mg of dietary iron a day, which balances the iron lost through shed intestinal mucosal cells, menstruation, and other blood loss. Regulation of the absorption of dietary iron from the duodenum plays a critical role in iron homeostasis [15]. Most of the dietary iron is absorbed at the apical surface of duodenal enterocytes. Iron released into the circulation then binds to transferrin, which has two binding sites for one atom of iron each; about 30–40 % of these sites are occupied in normal physiological conditions. Transferrin carrying iron interacts with specific surface receptors (transferrin-receptor 1, TfR1) to form transferrin-receptor complexes that are endocytosed into the target cells. Erythroid precursors express high levels of TfR1 to ensure the uptake of iron.

Iron homeostasis can be disturbed by inflammation. Activation of the immune and inflammatory systems inhibits iron absorption and iron recirculation and increases ferritin synthesis and iron storage [16]. These effects lead to hypoferremia, iron-restricted erythropoiesis, and finally to mild to moderate anemia [17, 18].

Theoretically, vitamin B12 and folate deficiency may play a role in the development of anemia in ICU patients. However, the few data that are available suggest that these vitamins do not limit RBC production in most anemic critically ill patients [19].

2.4.2   Inappropriately Low Circulating Erythropoietin Concentrations

The normal response to anemia is an increase in EPO release from the kidneys. Values of circulating EPO concentrations have been established in otherwise healthy patients with various degrees of anemia [7]. Using these data as references for an appropriate response to anemia, many studies have shown that critically ill patients have inappropriately low EPO concentrations for their degree of anemia [20, 21]. The blunted EPO response during critical illness probably results from inhibition of the EPO gene by inflammatory cytokines [22, 23].

2.5   Abnormal RBC Maturation

Critical illness is often associated with increased concentrations of inflammatory cytokines, such as tumor necrosis factor (TNF)-α, interleukin (IL)-1, and IL-6, particularly during sepsis. Many of these cytokines have been shown to directly inhibit RBC formation. Other circulating factors, such as interferon-γ, have been shown to induce apoptosis of erythroid precursors in experimental studies. In addition to the relative deficiency of circulating EPO and decreased iron availability, these factors help explain the poor erythroid response to anemia in critically ill patients. Bone marrow hyporeactivity is also suggested by the fact that reticulocyte counts are usually not increased in anemic critically ill patients unless pharmacological doses of EPO are being administered to stimulate erythropoiesis [19, 24].

2.6   Reduced Red Cell Survival

In healthy humans, erythrocytes have a lifespan of approximately 100–120 days. Normal RBC aging leads to changes in membrane characteristics with decreased deformability, loss of volume and surface area, increased cell density and viscosity, and alterations in the intracellular milieu [13]. These changes result in a decrease in cellular energy levels, increased hemoglobin-oxygen affinity, reduced ability to repair oxidant injury, and decreased ability of the cells to deform when passing through the microvasculature [25]. These changes also indicate that the RBCs are ready for removal by the spleen and reticuloendothelial system. Other determinants of RBC survival include the premature death of mature RBCs (eryptosis) and the removal of RBCs just released from the marrow (neocytolysis). Eryptosis, an apoptosis-like process, is thought to be, in part, triggered by excessive oxidant RBC injury and is inhibited by EPO, which therefore prolongs the lifespan of circulating RBCs [26]. Excessive eryptosis may lead to the development of anemia [27]. Neocytolysis is a process initiated by a sudden decrease in EPO levels by which young circulating RBCs are selectively removed from the circulation [28]. Eryptosis and neocytolysis act at different points in the lifespan of the RBC and thus provide a flexible means of controlling the regulation of total RBC mass.

The normal aging alterations in RBC rheology may occur earlier in critically ill patients, which may have clinical implications [29]. It is likely that critical illness and sepsis, in particular, reduce RBC lifespan, but there is as yet no direct evidence to support this. Experimental data have shown that inflammatory mediators, such as TNF-α and IL-1, can decrease erythrocyte survival time in other settings [30], and oxidative stress has been shown to induce premature apoptosis in RBCs [31].

2.7   Increased RBC Destruction

Hemolysis may be associated with several pathologic conditions, including hemoglobinopathies, hemolytic anemias, bacterial infections, malaria, and trauma. Hemolysis can also occur in conditions in which mechanical forces can lead to RBC rupture, such as surgical procedures, hemodialysis, and blood transfusion. Extracorporeal circuits may lead to complete RBC destruction or cause less severe damage resulting in altered rheological properties. Hemolysis results in release of free plasma hemoglobin and heme, which are toxic to the vascular endothelium [32]. Although most RBC destruction in standard cardiopulmonary bypass procedures can be managed by the endogenous clearing mechanisms, in some cases, for example, in extensive surgery and with prolonged support, higher degrees of hemolysis may occur, and levels of plasma free hemoglobin can rise substantially. These patients are especially susceptible to the toxic influence of un-scavenged RBC constituents and the loss of RBC rheological properties [33].

Hypersplenism may also lead to excessive RBC destruction and is characterized by a significant reduction in one or more of the cellular elements of the blood in the presence of normocellular or hypercellular bone marrow and splenomegaly [34]. In patients with chronic liver disease, hypersplenism secondary to portal hypertension is an important cause of anemia. The main characteristics of hypersplenism are related to the presence of pancytopenia; hemolytic anemia occurs because of intrasplenic destruction of erythrocytes [35].

2.8   Hemodilution

Critically ill patients frequently develop intravascular hypovolemia requiring fluid resuscitation. Current management involves administering crystalloid or colloid solutions during resuscitation and withholding RBC transfusion unless there is severe hemorrhage. The resultant relatively modest hemodilution contributes to the rapid decrease in hemoglobin concentrations seen early after ICU admission in many critically ill patients [36] and can cause anemia without decreasing RBC mass.

2.9   Conclusion

Anemia is a common occurrence in critically ill patients and is associated with considerable morbidity and worse outcomes. The etiology of anemia in individual patients is commonly multifactorial. Understanding the possible etiologic factors of anemia is crucial to prevent its occurrence and identify the appropriate therapeutic approach to treat this condition in critically ill patients.

References

1. Vincent JL, Baron JF, Reinhart K, Gattinoni L, Thijs L, et al. Anemia and blood transfusion in critically ill patients. JAMA. 2002;288:1499–507.
2. Corwin HL, Gettinger A, Pearl RG, Fink MP, Levy MM, et al. The CRIT Study: Anemia and blood transfusion in the critically ill – current clinical practice in the United States. Crit Care Med. 2004;32:39–52.
3. Vincent JL, Sakr Y, Creteur J. Anemia in the intensive care unit. Can J Anaesth. 2003;50:S53–9.

4. Chohan SS, McArdle F, McClelland DB, Mackenzie SJ, Walsh TS. Red cell transfusion practice following the transfusion requirements in critical care (TRICC) study: prospective observational cohort study in a large UK intensive care unit. Vox Sang. 2003;84:211–8.
5. Walsh TS, Saleh EE, Lee RJ, McClelland DB. The prevalence and characteristics of anaemia at discharge home after intensive care. Intensive Care Med. 2006;32:1206–13.
6. Weiss G, Goodnough LT. Anemia of chronic disease. N Engl J Med. 2005;352:1011–23.
7. Beguin Y, Clemons GK, Pootrakul P, Fillet G. Quantitative assessment of erythropoiesis and functional classification of anemia based on measurements of serum transferrin receptor and erythropoietin. Blood. 1993;81:1067–76.
8. Smoller BR, Kruskall MS. Phlebotomy for diagnostic laboratory tests in adults. Pattern of use and effect on transfusion requirements. N Engl J Med. 1986;314:1233–5.
9. Branco BC, Inaba K, Doughty R, Brooks J, Barmparas G, et al. The increasing burden of phlebotomy in the development of anaemia and need for blood transfusion amongst trauma patients. Injury. 2012;43:78–83.
10. Cook D, Heyland D, Griffith L, Cook R, Marshall J, et al. Risk factors for clinically important upper gastrointestinal bleeding in patients requiring mechanical ventilation. Canadian Critical Care Trials Group. Crit Care Med. 1999;27:2812–7.
11. Westbrook A, Pettila V, Nichol A, Bailey MJ, Syres G, et al. Transfusion practice and guidelines in Australian and New Zealand intensive care units. Intensive Care M ed. 2010;36:1138–46.
12. Sinclair AM. Erythropoiesis stimulating agents: approaches to modulate activity. Biologics. 2013;7:161–74.
13. Hayden SJ, Albert TJ, Watkins TR, Swenson ER. Anemia in critical illness: insights into etiology, consequences, and management. Am J Respir Crit Care Med. 2012;185:1049–57.
14. Hillman RS, Henderson PA. Control of marrow production by the level of iron supply. J Clin Invest. 1969;48:454–60.
15. Andrews NC. Forging a field: the golden age of iron biology. Blood. 2008;112:219–30.
16. Munoz M, Villar I, Garcia-Erce JA. An update on iron physiology. World J Gastroenterol. 2009;15:4617–26.
17. Franke A, Lante W, Fackeldey V, Becker HP, Kurig E, et al. Pro-inflammatory cytokines after different kinds of cardio-thoracic surgical procedures: is what we see what we know? Eur J Cardiothorac Surg. 2005;28:569–75.
18. Cook JD. Diagnosis and management of iron-deficiency anaemia. Best Pract Res Clin Haematol. 2005;18:319–32.
19. Rodriguez RM, Corwin HL, Gettinger A, Corwin MJ, Gubler D, et al. Nutritional deficiencies and blunted erythropoietin response as causes of the anemia of critical illness. J Crit Care. 2001;16:36–41.
20. Rogiers P, Zhang H, Leeman M, Nagler J, Neels H, et al. Erythropoietin response is blunted in critically ill patients. Intensive Care Med. 1997;23:159–62.
21. Elliot JM, Virankabutra T, Jones S, Tanudsintum S, Lipkin G, et al. Erythropoietin mimics the acute phase response in critical illness. Crit Care. 2003;7:R35–40.
22. Jelkmann W, Pagel H, Wolff M, Fandrey J. Monokines inhibiting erythropoietin production in human hepatoma cultures and in isolated perfused rat kidneys. Life Sci. 1992;50:301–8.
23. Corwin HL, Krantz SB. Anemia of the critically ill: "acute" anemia of chronic disease. Crit Care Med. 2000;28:3098–9.
24. van Iperen CE, Gaillard CA, Kraaijenhagen RJ, Braam BG, Marx JJ, et al. Response of erythropoiesis and iron metabolism to recombinant human erythropoietin in intensive care unit patients. Crit Care Med. 2000;28:2773–8.
25. Ott P. Membrane acetylcholinesterases: purification, molecular properties and interactions with amphiphilic environments. Biochim Biophys Acta. 1985;822:375–92.
26. Myssina S, Huber SM, Birka C, Lang PA, Lang KS, et al. Inhibition of erythrocyte cation channels by erythropoietin. J Am Soc Nephrol. 2003;14:2750–7.
27. Lang F, Lang KS, Lang PA, Huber SM, Wieder T. Mechanisms and significance of eryptosis. Antioxid Redox Signal. 2006;8:1183–92.
28. Rice L, Alfrey CP. The negative regulation of red cell mass by neocytolysis: physiologic and pathophysiologic manifestations. Cell Physiol Biochem. 2005;15:245–50.

29. Reggiori G, Occhipinti G, De GA, Vincent JL, Piagnerelli M. Early alterations of red blood cell rheology in critically ill patients. Crit Care Med. 2009;37:3041–6.
30. Scharte M, Fink MP. Red blood cell physiology in critical illness. Crit Care Med. 2003;31:S651–7.
31. Lang KS, Duranton C, Poehlmann H, Myssina S, Bauer C, et al. Cation channels trigger apoptotic death of erythrocytes. Cell Death Differ. 2003;10:249–56.
32. Vinchi F, Tolosano E. Therapeutic approaches to limit hemolysis-driven endothelial dysfunction: scavenging free heme to preserve vasculature homeostasis. Oxid Med Cell Longev. 2013;2013:396527.
33. Vercaemst L. Hemolysis in cardiac surgery patients undergoing cardiopulmonary bypass: a review in search of a treatment algorithm. J Extra Corpor Technol. 2008;40:257–67.
34. Jeker R. Hypersplenism. Ther Umsch. 2013;70:152–6.
35. Gonzalez-Casas R, Jones EA, Moreno-Otero R. Spectrum of anemia associated with chronic liver disease. World J Gastroenterol. 2009;15:4653–8.
36. Van PY, Riha GM, Cho SD, Underwood SJ, Hamilton GJ, et al. Blood volume analysis can distinguish true anemia from hemodilution in critically ill patients. J Trauma. 2011;70:646–51.

Jean-Louis Vincent

Abstract

Blood transfusions are a relatively common event in patients with sepsis. Although severe anemia is associated with worse outcomes, hemoglobin levels less than the classically quoted 10 g/dl are well tolerated in many patients, and it is difficult to determine whether or when such patients should be transfused. Importantly, there can be no one transfusion trigger or threshold for all patients, rather the benefit/risk ratio of transfusion should be assessed in each patient taking into account multiple factors including physiological variables, age, disease severity, and coexisting cardiac ischemia. The ultimate goal of transfusion is to improve tissue oxygenation, but our ability to measure these changes and hence determine the need for and response to transfusion is still limited.

3.1 Introduction

Patients with sepsis make up a large proportion of the intensive care unit (ICU) population, and although outcomes have improved over the last decade [1], these patients, particularly those with septic shock, still have mortality rates in the region of 20–30 % [2, 3]. There are no effective specific antisepsis treatments, and management of patients with sepsis thus relies largely on early recognition allowing timely administration of appropriate antibiotics, suitable source control measures, and effective resuscitation strategies. The aims of resuscitation are essentially to restore and maintain tissue oxygen delivery (DO_2) so that organs can function optimally.

There are various means by which DO_2 can be improved, including fluid administration, vasopressor agents to restore perfusion pressure, and inotropic agents to

J.-L. Vincent
Department of Intensive Care, Erasme University Hospital, Université libre de Bruxelles,
Route de Lennik 808, B-1070 Brussels, Belgium
e-mail: jlvincen@ulb.ac.be

© Springer International Publishing Switzerland 2015
N.P. Juffermans, T.S. Walsh (eds.), *Transfusion in the Intensive Care Unit*,
DOI 10.1007/978-3-319-08735-1_3

support cardiac function and increase cardiac output. Blood transfusions have also been widely used as a means of improving tissue DO_2, although this relationship is not straightforward. Indeed, the increased blood viscosity as a result of the transfusion can lead to a decrease in cardiac output (CO) and hence in DO_2 [4], except in conditions of hemorrhage and hemodilution in which increased viscosity can improve microcirculatory flow and hence DO_2 [5]. As many as 30 % of intensive care unit (ICU) patients receive a transfusion at some point during their ICU stay [6–11], but there is still considerable debate about the benefit/risk ratio of this intervention and when or if any individual patient should be transfused.

In this chapter, we will review the balance between DO_2 and oxygen uptake (VO_2) in sepsis and the effects of red blood cell transfusion on this balance and discuss some of the more recent trials that have investigated hemoglobin levels and the beneficial and adverse effects of transfusion in critically ill patients.

3.2   Oxygen Delivery and Consumption in Sepsis

Tissue oxygenation essentially relies on DO_2, VO_2, and the ability of the tissue to extract oxygen. DO_2 is the rate at which oxygen is transported from the lungs to the tissues and is the product of the CO and the arterial oxygen content (CaO_2): $DO_2 = CO \times CaO_2$, where CaO_2 = hemoglobin concentration (Hb) $\times$ arterial oxygen saturation (SaO_2) $\times 1.34$ (the oxygen carrying capacity of Hb). DO_2 can, therefore, be influenced by changes in CO, hemoglobin concentration, and oxygen saturation. VO_2 is the amount of oxygen removed from the blood by the tissues per minute and is the product of the CO and the difference between CaO_2 and mixed venous oxygen content (CvO_2): $VO_2 = CO \times (CaO_2 - CvO_2)$. VO_2 is determined by the metabolic rate of the tissues, which increases during physical activity, hyperthermia, shivering, etc. The ratio of the oxygen consumed to that delivered (VO_2/DO_2) represents the amount of oxygen extracted by the tissues, the oxygen extraction ratio (O_2ER).

As tissues are unable to store oxygen, it is important for them to have a system by which delivery of oxygen can be adjusted efficiently to oxygen demands. Under normal physiological conditions, as DO_2 decreases, oxygen extraction increases to compensate and maintain VO_2, ensuring adequate tissue oxygenation for aerobic metabolism and normal cellular function: VO_2 is independent of DO_2. Indeed, at rest, VO_2 is only about 25 % of DO_2, so that there is a large reserve of oxygen available for extraction if needed as DO_2 falls [12]. However, a point is reached at which oxygen extraction is unable to increase further and a so-called critical DO_2 is attained at which VO_2 becomes dependent on DO_2; any further decrease in DO_2 is associated with a decrease in VO_2 and anaerobic metabolism with a rise in blood lactate levels [13–15].

During septic shock, the ability of tissues to extract oxygen is reduced so that this VO_2/DO_2 relationship can be altered with the critical DO_2 set at higher values such that VO_2 is dependent on DO_2 over a larger range of values [13–15]. The reasons for the reduced oxygen extraction abilities in sepsis have not been fully elucidated but are likely to be related in part to the microcirculatory changes seen in sepsis, including increased heterogeneity, increased stop-flow capillaries, and increased shunting of DO_2 from arterioles to venules [12]. Impaired ability of mitochondria to use the available oxygen may also play a role in microcirculatory dysoxia [16].

3.3   Anemia in Sepsis

Anemia, widely defined in ICU studies as a hemoglobin level <12 g/dl [7, 17], is common in critically ill patients [6, 7, 18]. In the ABC study [3], 29 % of patients had a hemoglobin concentration <10 g/dl on admission. In a Scottish cohort, 25 % of patients had a hemoglobin concentration <9 g/dl on ICU admission [19]. Hemoglobin concentrations decrease during the ICU stay, particularly in septic patients, in whom Nguyen et al. [20] reported a decrease of 0.68 ± 0.66 g/dl/day; this study also noted that hemoglobin concentrations continued to decrease after the third day in patients with sepsis but not in those without [20].

Multiple factors act together to cause anemia in the critically ill patient, including primary blood losses (trauma, surgery, gastrointestinal bleeding, etc.), phlebotomy losses, which can reach as much as 40 ml/day [20], hemodilution secondary to fluid resuscitation, blunted erythropoietin (EPO) production, abnormalities in iron metabolism, and altered red blood cell production and maturation [21–23]. In healthy subjects, compensatory mechanisms, including the increased oxygen extraction discussed above, but also reflex increases in CO because of decreased blood viscosity, increased adrenergic response, causing tachycardia and increased myocardial contractility, and blood flow redistribution (to heart and brain) enable severe anemia to be tolerated [24]. However, in critically ill patients, compensatory mechanisms are less efficient, and oxygen reserves are reduced so that lesser degrees of anemia may have greater consequences on organ function and outcome. Oddo et al., in a retrospective study of patients with traumatic brain injury who had had brain tissue oxygen tension ($PbtO_2$) measured, noted that anemia associated with reduced $PbtO_2$ was a risk factor for unfavorable outcome, but not anemia alone [25]. Patients with myocardial ischemic disease may be particularly sensitive to the effects of anemia because the associated tachycardia and increased contractility may increase myocardial oxygen demand, which will need to be met by increased coronary blood flow as myocardial oxygen extraction is almost maximal already at rest [23, 26].

3.4   Monitoring VO_2/DO_2 and Tissue Oxygenation During Transfusion

Because DO_2 is the product of CO and CaO_2 is determined in part by the hemoglobin concentration, when the hemoglobin concentration decreases, DO_2 will decrease (if CO remains unchanged). Hence, one may anticipate that increasing the hemoglobin by giving a transfusion would help increase DO_2 as has indeed been shown in several studies [27–29]; although by increasing blood viscosity, some of the compensatory mechanisms of acute anemia on left ventricular pre- and afterload will be reduced, thus limiting the effects on DO_2 [5]. Moreover, even if DO_2 does increase, there is no guarantee that VO_2 and hence oxygen availability to the tissues will also increase, particularly in patients with an abnormal VO_2/DO_2 relationship and an altered microcirculation, such as those with sepsis [27, 29, 30]. There are several possible reasons for this including the fact that the ability of hemoglobin to download oxygen may be altered in sepsis because of microcirculatory changes, such as altered red blood cell deformability, altered oxygen extraction capabilities, reduced functional capillary density, and increased heterogeneity of flow. The ability of hemoglobin to deliver oxygen may also be influenced by changes that occur during storage of blood [31] and by increased blood viscosity following transfusion leading to reduced microcirculatory flow. Additionally, tissue oxygen demands are increased in patients with sepsis.

Importantly, different tissues have different critical DO_2 values and VO_2/DO_2 relationships and develop hypoxia at different degrees of acute anemia [32]. Hence, global assessment of the VO_2/DO_2 relationship cannot be used to guide therapy. "Coupling of data," which occurs when both variables have been calculated from the same values, is also a problem when using this relationship [15]. Cardiac output represents total body blood flow and can be monitored almost continuously but offers no information on regional organ perfusion. Cardiac output is also highly variable among individuals and varies according to oxygen requirements; for example, in sepsis the typically "normal" or high CO seen may be insufficient because of increased sepsis-related tissue oxygen requirements.

Mixed venous oxygen saturation (SvO_2) has been widely used as a marker of tissue oxygenation, and, indeed, as oxygen extraction increases to meet oxygen demands, SvO_2 will decrease. However, although low SvO_2 indicates poor tissue oxygenation, normal or high SvO_2 values do not necessarily mean that tissue oxygenation is adequate; for example, if a tissue is unable to extract oxygen, the venous return from that area may still have a high oxygen content although the tissues may be hypoxic. Central venous oxygen saturation ($ScvO_2$) is increasingly used as a less invasive surrogate for SvO_2, but again this is a global measure. Rivers et al. [33], in their landmark study, randomized patients admitted to an emergency department with severe sepsis and septic shock to receive standard therapy (targeted at a central venous pressure [CVP] of 8–12 mmHg, mean arterial pressure [MAP] ≥ 65 mmHg, and urine output ≥ 0.5 ml/kg/h) or to the so-called early goal-directed therapy (EGDT) in which an $ScvO_2$ of at least 70 % was also targeted by optimizing fluid administration, giving blood transfusions to maintain hematocrit ≥ 30 %, and/ or giving dobutamine to a maximum of 20 μg/kg/min. The EGDT group received more fluids, and more were treated with dobutamine; the number of transfused patients was also greater than in the standard therapy group. Patients in the EGDT group had significantly lower mortality rates than other patients, and this study therefore seemed to support the use of $ScvO_2$ values to guide therapy, including transfusions [33]. However, in the recently published Protocolized Care for Early

Septic Shock (ProCESS) study [34], there were no significant differences in 90-day mortality, 1-year mortality, or the need for organ support in patients managed with protocolized EGDT – using a similar protocol to that used by Rivers et al., protocolized standard therapy or usual care.

The O_2ER is easy to calculate, and plotting cardiac index (CI) against O_2ER and relating them to isopleths of VO_2 can help identify whether a patient has reached the point of VO_2/DO_2 dependency and evaluate the adequacy of CO in complex patients [35]. In patients with anemia and normal cardiac function, a CI/O_2ER ratio <10 suggests an inadequate CI that is likely due to hypovolemia [35].

As tissue oxygenation becomes inadequate, anaerobic metabolism begins to take over from aerobic metabolism and blood lactate levels rise. Although other factors can also result in increased blood lactate levels [36], a blood lactate level greater than 2 mEq/l suggests inadequate tissue perfusion and oxygenation. Hyperlactatemia is associated with a poor prognosis in critically ill patients in general and in those with sepsis [37]. As with many other measures, trends in lactate levels are of greater value than any individual value [38].

There is no ideal measure for determining optimal tissue oxygenation, and adequacy of DO_2 must be assessed using a combination of the above variables along with clinical examination.

3.5   Microcirculatory Effects of Blood Transfusions

With the advent of new techniques to monitor the microcirculation, several studies have now reported the effects of transfusion on the microcirculation in human subjects. In a small early study using orthogonal polarization spectral (OPS) imaging, Genzel-Boroviczény et al. reported an improvement in functional capillary density following transfusion in anemic preterm infants, indicating improved microvascular perfusion [39]. In patients undergoing on-pump cardiac surgery, Yuruk and colleagues [40] reported, using sidestream dark-field (SDF) imaging, that blood transfusion was associated with microcirculatory recruitment resulting in increased capillary density, thus reducing the oxygen diffusion distance to the cells. Using near-infrared spectroscopy (NIRS), the same authors reported that transfusion increased thenar and sublingual tissue oxygen saturation (StO_2) and thenar and sublingual tissue hemoglobin index (THI) in outpatients with chronic anemia [41]. In critically ill patients, Creteur et al., using the same NIRS technique, noted that blood transfusion was not associated with changes in muscle tissue oxygenation, VO_2, or microvascular reactivity in all patients, but that muscle VO_2 and microvascular reactivity did improve in patients in whom these variables were altered prior to the transfusion [42]. Similar findings have been made in patients with severe sepsis [43, 44] and trauma [45]. In a retrospective study of patients with severe sepsis who had a microdialysis catheter inserted for interstitial fluid measurements, blood transfusion was associated with a decrease in the interstitial lactate/pyruvate ratio, and these changes were again correlated with the pre-transfusion lactate/pyruvate ratio [46].

Studies have also assessed the impact of transfusion of fresh versus stored blood cell units on the microcirculation. In healthy volunteers, there were no differences in sublingual OPS-derived microcirculatory variables or NIRS-derived StO_2 after transfusion with 7-day or 42-day stored blood [47]. Walsh et al. reported no difference between stored (>20 days) and fresh (<5 days) cells on gastric tonometry indices in anemic critically ill patients [48], but Weinberg et al. reported a decrease in NIRS StO_2 and sidestream dark-field (SDF) capillary vascular density with transfusion of older units in trauma patients [49]. Some of the negative effects of blood transfusion may be due to the presence of leukocytes, and it has been proposed that use of leukodepleted blood should be preferred in critically ill patients. A recent pilot study in which 20 patients with sepsis were randomized to receive either leukode-pleted or non-leukodepleted blood showed no clear superiority of leukodepleted over non-leukodepleted blood although leukodepleted blood was associated with more favorable changes in MFI and blood flow velocity [50].

3.6 Putting the Theory into Practice: Clinical Trials of Transfusion Triggers in Septic Patients

We have seen that blood transfusion can improve DO_2 but may not directly help improve tissue oxygenation. Patients with sepsis frequently develop anemia [20], which is known to be associated with worse outcomes in critically ill patients [11, 51, 52], but are blood transfusions actually of benefit? When should critically ill patients with sepsis be transfused? Several early observational studies suggested worse outcomes in critically ill patients who received a transfusion compared to those who did not [6, 7], casting doubt on the supposed benefits of transfusion, but more recent studies have suggested the opposite [8, 11]. Some of these differences may be related to the timing of transfusion as benefits are likely to be greatest in the early stages of disease than in later phases when patients are stable or already have established organ failure [53]. Indeed, the Surviving Sepsis Campaign guidelines give different recommendations based on the duration of the septic episode: during the first 6 h of resuscitation, they suggest that transfusion should be given to maintain the hematocrit above 30 % if $ScvO_2$ remains below 70 % despite initial fluid and vasopressor therapy; this recommendation was, however, largely based on the Rivers study [33], so may need to be reconsidered in light of the ProCESS results [34]. After this initial period, the SSC guidelines recommend transfusion when the hemoglobin concentration is less than 7.0 g/dl to maintain a concentration of 7.0–9.0 g/dl (grade 1B). In certain circumstances, such as severe hypoxemia, ischemic coronary artery disease, or acute hemorrhage, higher thresholds may be warranted [54]. Guidelines from the British Committee for Standards in Hematology make similar recommendations [55].

The Transfusion Requirements in Critical Care (TRICC) study published in 1999 [56] changed many intensivists' conceptions of blood transfusion, and physicians worldwide began to reconsider their transfusion thresholds [57], although one recent study suggested that transfusion rates only decreased in high-volume ICUs

(>200 admissions per year) but continued to increase in low-volume hospitals [58]. Importantly, much has changed in intensive care since 1994–1997 when the TRICC study was conducted. Blood transfusion medicine has evolved so that blood transfusions are now safer. The general process of care has improved, and patients are being diagnosed and treated more rapidly with appropriate and effective resuscitation. So what new evidence is available on transfusion thresholds? There have been no large-scale studies comparing one transfusion trigger with another in a general population of critically ill patients since the TRICC study, and there are few specific data in septic patients. But there have been several studies comparing different thresholds in other groups of patients. A randomized controlled study in more than 500 patients undergoing cardiac surgery with cardiopulmonary bypass reported that a perioperative restrictive transfusion strategy (to maintain a hematocrit at least 24 %) was associated with similar morbidity/mortality outcomes compared to a more liberal strategy (to maintain a hematocrit of at least 30 %) [59]. In addition, regardless of the transfusion strategy, the number of transfused red blood cell units was an independent risk factor for clinical complications or death at 30 days (hazard ratio 1.21 for each additional unit transfused; 95 % confidence interval 1.1–1.4, $P = .002$). In a recent pilot study that included 100 elderly (>55 years), mechanically ventilated ICU patients, there was a trend to reduced mortality in patients managed using a restrictive (hemoglobin threshold 7.0 g/dl) compared to a more liberal (9.0 g/dl) strategy [60]. In a small randomized study in 44 patients with subarachnoid hemorrhage and high risk of vasospasm, Naidech et al. [61] reported that targeting a higher hemoglobin concentration (11.5 g/dl) was as safe as targeting a lower hemoglobin level (10 g/dl) and may have reduced the incidence of cortical cerebral infarction. In a randomized study of 2,016 patients ≥50 years of age with a history of or risk factors for cardiovascular disease after hip fracture surgery, a liberal transfusion strategy (hemoglobin threshold 10 g/dl) was not associated with reduced mortality or function at 60 days compared with a restrictive strategy (symptoms of anemia or physician discretion for a hemoglobin level of <8 g/dl) [62].

3.7 Conclusion

Anemia is common in the critically ill patient and is associated with worse outcomes. Nevertheless, most patients can tolerate a degree of anemia, and it is difficult to determine whether or when such patients should be transfused. Strategies to reduce the development of anemia should be employed, including minimizing iatrogenic blood loss and oxygen consumption. Exogenous erythropoietin, iron, and Hb-based oxygen carriers may have a place in some patients, but further study is needed to determine their role.

Microcirculatory "shunting" can create local hypoxia even if global oxygenation parameters are normal, and strategies that act directly on regional perfusion or cellular metabolism are likely to be more effective than strategies aimed at increasing global DO_2. Transfusions seem to improve microcirculatory parameters in patients in whom these variables are altered prior to transfusion, and further study is needed to determine whether such variables could be used to guide transfusion. Current guidelines suggest targeting a hematocrit of >30 % in the early phase of sepsis [54], but this threshold should be assessed on an individual basis taking into account multiple factors including physiological variables, age, and coexisting cardiac ischemia [63, 64].

A study comparing a restrictive (at hemoglobin ≤7 g/dl) versus liberal (at hemoglobin ≤9 g/dl) transfusion protocol in patients with septic shock is currently ongoing (Transfusion Requirements in Septic Shock [TRISS] trial) [65] and may help provide additional guidance when considering transfusing patients with sepsis.

References

1. Kaukonen KM, Bailey M, Suzuki S, Pilcher D, Bellomo R. Mortality related to severe sepsis and septic shock among critically ill patients in Australia and New Zealand, 2000–2012. JAMA. 2014;311:1308–16.
2. Vincent JL, Marshall JC, Namendys-Silva SA, François B, Martin-Loeches I, Lipman J, Reinhart K, Antonelli M, Pickkers P, Njimi H, Jimenez E, Sakr Y. Assessment of the worldwide burden of critical illness: the Intensive Care Over Nations (ICON) audit. Lancet Respir Med. 2014;2:380–6.
3. Vincent JL, Rello J, Marshall J, Silva E, Anzueto A, Martin CD, Moreno R, Lipman J, Gomersall C, Sakr Y, Reinhart K. International study of the prevalence and outcomes of infection in intensive care units. JAMA. 2009;302:2323–9.
4. Martini J, Carpentier B, Negrete AC, Frangos JA, Intaglietta M. Paradoxical hypotension following increased hematocrit and blood viscosity. Am J Physiol Heart Circ Physiol. 2005;289:H2136–43.
5. Tsai AG, Hofmann A, Cabrales P, Intaglietta M. Perfusion vs. oxygen delivery in transfusion with "fresh" and "old" red blood cells: the experimental evidence. Transfus Apher Sci. 2010;43:69–78.
6. Vincent JL, Baron JF, Reinhart K, Gattinoni L, Thijs L, Webb A, Meier-Hellmann A, Nollet G, Peres-Bota D. Anemia and blood transfusion in critically ill patients. JAMA. 2002;288:1499–507.
7. Corwin HL, Gettinger A, Pearl RG, Fink MP, Levy MM, Abraham E, MacIntyre NR, Shabot MM, Duh MS, Shapiro MJ. The CRIT Study: Anemia and blood transfusion in the critically ill – current clinical practice in the United States. Crit Care Med. 2004;32:39–52.
8. Vincent JL, Sakr Y, Sprung C, Harboe S, Damas P. Are blood transfusions associated with greater mortality rates? Results of the Sepsis Occurrence in Acutely Ill Patients study. Anesthesiology. 2008;108:31–9.
9. Brophy DF, Harpe SE, Carl DE, Brophy GM. An epidemiological study of anemia and renal dysfunction in patients admitted to ICUs across the United States. Anemia. 2012;2012:938140.
10. Surgenor SD, Kramer RS, Olmstead EM, Ross CS, Sellke FW, Likosky DS, Marrin CA, Helm Jr RE, Leavitt BJ, Morton JR, Charlesworth DC, Clough RA, Hernandez F, Frumiento C, Benak A, DioData C, O'Connor GT. The association of perioperative red blood cell transfusions and decreased long-term survival after cardiac surgery. Anesth Analg. 2009;108:1741–6.
11. Sakr Y, Lobo S, Knuepfer S, Esser E, Bauer M, Settmacher U, Barz D, Reinhart K. Anemia and blood transfusion in a surgical intensive care unit. Crit Care. 2010;14:R92.
12. Kanoore Edul V, Dubin A, Ince C. The microcirculation as a therapeutic target in the treatment of sepsis and shock. Semin Respir Crit Care Med. 2011;32:558–68.
13. Squara P. Matching total body oxygen consumption and delivery: a crucial objective? Intensive Care Med. 2004;30:2170–9.

14. Vincent JL. DO$_2$/VO$_2$ relationships. In: Pinsky MR, Payen D, editors. Functional hemodynamic monitoring. Heidelberg: Springer; 2005. p. 251–8.

15. Leach RM, Treacher DF. The pulmonary physician in critical care * 2: oxygen delivery and consumption in the critically ill. Thorax. 2002;57:170–7.

16. Fink MP. Cytopathic hypoxia. Is oxygen use impaired in sepsis as a result of an acquired intrinsic derangement in cellular respiration? Crit Care Clin. 2002;18:165–75.

17. Hayden SJ, Albert TJ, Watkins TR, Swenson ER. Anemia in critical illness: insights into etiology, consequences, and management. Am J Respir Crit Care Med. 2012;185:1049–57.

18. Thomas J, Jensen L, Nahirniak S, Gibney RT. Anemia and blood transfusion practices in the critically ill: a prospective cohort review. Heart Lung. 2010;39:217–25.

19. Walsh TS, Lee RJ, Maciver CR, Garrioch M, MacKirdy F, Binning AR, Cole S, McClelland DB. Anemia during and at discharge from intensive care: the impact of restrictive blood transfusion practice. Intensive Care Med. 2006;32:100–9.

20. Nguyen BV, Bota DP, Melot C, Vincent JL. Time course of hemoglobin concentrations in nonbleeding intensive care unit patients. Crit Care Med. 2003;31:406–10.

21. Piagnerelli M, Zouaoui Boudjeltia K, Gulbis B, Vanhaeverbeek M, Vincent JL. Anemia in sepsis: the importance of red blood cell membrane changes. Transfus Altern Transfus Med. 2007;9:143–9.

22. Vincent JL, Sakr Y, Creteur J. Anemia in the intensive care unit. Can J Anaesth. 2003;50:S53–9.

23. Lelubre C, Vincent JL. Red blood cell transfusion in the critically ill patient. Ann Intensive Care. 2011;1:43.

24. Weiskopf RB, Viele MK, Feiner J, Kelley S, Lieberman J, Noorani M, Leung JM, Fisher DM, Murray WR, Toy P, Moore MA. Human cardiovascular and metabolic response to acute, severe isovolemic anemia. JAMA. 1998;279:217–21.

25. Oddo M, Levine JM, Kumar M, Iglesias K, Frangos S, Maloney-Wilensky E, Le Roux PD. Anemia and brain oxygen after severe traumatic brain injury. Intensive Care Med. 2012;38:1497–504.

26. Levy PS, Kim SJ, Eckel PK, Chavez R, Ismail EF, Gould SA, Ramez SM, Crystal GJ. Limit to cardiac compensation during acute isovolemic hemodilution: influence of coronary stenosis. Am J Physiol. 1993;265:H340–9.

27. Lorente JA, Landin L, De Pablo R, Renes E, Rodriguez-Diaz R, Liste D. Effects of blood transfusion on oxygen transport variables in severe sepsis. Crit Care Med. 1993;21:1312–8.

28. Casutt M, Seifert B, Pasch T, Schmid ER, Turina MI, Spahn DR. Factors influencing the individual effects of blood transfusions on oxygen delivery and oxygen consumption. Crit Care Med. 1999;27:2194–200.

29. Suttner S, Piper SN, Kumle B, Lang K, Rohm KD, Isgro F, Boldt J. The influence of allogeneic red blood cell transfusion compared with 100 % oxygen ventilation on systemic oxygen transport and skeletal muscle oxygen tension after cardiac surgery. Anesth Analg. 2004;99:2–11.

30. Fernandes Jr CJ, Akamine N, De Marco FV, De Souza JA, Lagudis S, Knobel E. Red blood cell transfusion does not increase oxygen consumption in critically ill septic patients. Crit Care. 2001;5:362–7.

31. Almac E, Ince C. The impact of storage on red cell function in blood transfusion. Best Pract Res Clin Anaesthesiol. 2007;21:195–208.

32. Lauscher P, Kertscho H, Schmidt O, Zimmermann R, Rosenberger P, Zacharowski K, Meier J. Determination of organ-specific anemia tolerance. Crit Care Med. 2013;41:1037–45.

33. Rivers E, Nguyen B, Havstad S, Ressler J, Muzzin A, Knoblich B, Peterson E, Tomlanovich M. Early goal-directed therapy in the treatment of severe sepsis and septic shock. N Engl J Med. 2001;345:1368–77.

34. The ProCESS Investigators. A randomized trial of protocol-based care for early septic shock. N Engl J Med. 2014;370:1683–93.

35. Yalavatti GS, DeBacker D, Vincent JL. Assessment of cardiac index in anemic patients. Chest. 2000;118:782–7.

36. De Backer D. Lactic acidosis. Minerva Anestesiol. 2003;69:281–4.

37. Mikkelsen ME, Miltiades AN, Gaieski DF, Goyal M, Fuchs BD, Shah CV, Bellamy SL, Christie JD. Serum lactate is associated with mortality in severe sepsis independent of organ failure and shock. Crit Care Med. 2009;37:1670–7.

38. Nichol A, Bailey M, Egi M, Pettila V, French C, Stachowski E, Reade MC, Cooper DJ, Bellomo R. Dynamic lactate indices as predictors of outcome in critically ill patients. Crit Care. 2011;15:R242.

39. Genzel-Boroviczeny O, Christ F, Glas V. Blood transfusion increases functional capillary density in the skin of anemic preterm infants. Pediatr Res. 2004;56:751–5.

40. Yuruk K, Almac E, Bezemer R, Goedhart P, de Mol B, Ince C. Blood transfusions recruit the microcirculation during cardiac surgery. Transfusion. 2011;51:961–7.

41. Yuruk K, Bartels SA, Milstein DM, Bezemer R, Biemond BJ, Ince C. Red blood cell transfusions and tissue oxygenation in anemic hematology outpatients. Transfusion. 2012;52:641–6.

42. Creteur J, Neves AP, Vincent JL. Near-infrared spectroscopy technique to evaluate the effects of red blood cell transfusion on tissue oxygenation. Crit Care. 2009;13 Suppl 5:S11.

43. Sakr Y, Chierego M, Piagnerelli M, Verdant C, Dubois MJ, Koch M, Creteur J, Gullo A, Vincent JL, De Backer D. Microvascular response to red blood cell transfusion in patients with severe sepsis. Crit Care Med. 2007;35:1639–44.

44. Sadaka F, Aggu-Sher R, Krause K, O'Brien J, Armbrecht ES, Taylor RW. The effect of red blood cell transfusion on tissue oxygenation and microcirculation in severe septic patients. Ann Intensive Care. 2011;1:46.

45. Weinberg JA, MacLennan PA, Vandromme-Cusick MJ, Angotti JM, Magnotti LJ, Kerby JD, Rue III LW, Barnum SR, Patel RP. Microvascular response to red blood cell transfusion in trauma patients. Shock. 2012;37:276–81.

46. Kopterides P, Theodorakopoulou M, Nikitas N, Ilias I, Vassiliadi DA, Orfanos SE, Tsangaris I, Maniatis NA, Tsantes AE, Travlou A, Dimitriadis G, Armaganidis A, Ungerstedt U, Dimopoulou I. Red blood cell transfusion affects microdialysis-assessed interstitial lactate/pyruvate ratio in critically ill patients with late sepsis. Intensive Care Med. 2012;38:1843–50.

47. Roberson RS, Lockhart E, Shapiro NI, Bandarenko N, McMahon TJ, Massey MJ, White WD, Bennett-Guerrero E. Impact of transfusion of autologous 7- versus 42-day-old AS-3 red blood cells on tissue oxygenation and the microcirculation in healthy volunteers. Transfusion. 2012;52:2459–64.

48. Walsh TS, McArdle F, McLellan SA, Maciver C, Maginnis M, Prescott RJ, McClelland DB. Does the storage time of transfused red blood cells influence regional or global indexes of tissue oxygenation in anemic critically ill patients? Crit Care Med. 2004;32:364–71.

49. Weinberg JA, MacLennan PA, Vandromme-Cusick MJ, Magnotti LJ, Kerby JD, Rue III LW, Angotti JM, Garrett CA, Hendrick LE, Croce MA, Fabian TC, Barnum SR, Patel RP. The deleterious effect of red blood cell storage on microvascular response to transfusion. J Trauma Acute Care Surg. 2013;75:807–12.

50. Donati A, Damiani E, Luchetti MM, Domizi R, Scorcella C, Carsetti A, Gabbanelli V, Carletti P, Bencivenga R, Vink H, Adrario E, Piagnerelli M, Gabrielli A, Pelaia P, Ince C. Microcirculatory effects of the transfusion of leukodepleted or non-leukodepleted red blood cells in septic patients: a pilot study. Crit Care. 2014;18:R33.

51. Mudumbai SC, Cronkite R, Hu KU, Wagner T, Hayashi K, Ozanne GM, Davies MF, Heidenreich P, Bertaccini E. Association of admission hematocrit with 6-month and 1-year mortality in intensive care unit patients. Transfusion. 2011;51:2148–59.

52. Koch CG, Li L, Sun Z, Hixson ED, Tang A, Phillips SC, Blackstone EH, Henderson JM. Hospital-acquired anemia: prevalence, outcomes, and healthcare implications. J Hosp Med. 2013;8:506–12.

53. Pape A, Stein P, Horn O, Habler O. Clinical evidence of blood transfusion effectiveness. Blood Transfus. 2009;7:250–8.

54. Dellinger RP, Levy MM, Rhodes A, Annane D, Gerlach H, Opal SM, Sevransky JE, Sprung CL, Douglas IS, Jaeschke R, Osborn TM, Nunnally ME, Townsend SR, Reinhart K, Kleinpell RM, Angus DC, Deutschman CS, Machado FR, Rubenfeld GD, Webb S, Beale RJ, Vincent JL, Moreno R. Surviving sepsis campaign: international guidelines for management of severe sepsis and septic shock, 2012. Intensive Care Med. 2013;39:165–228.

55. Retter A, Wyncoll D, Pearse R, Carson D, McKechnie S, Stanworth S, Allard S, Thomas D, Walsh T. Guidelines on the management of anaemia and red cell transfusion in adult critically ill patients. Br J Haematol. 2013;160:445–64.
56. Hebert PC, Wells G, Blajchman MA, Marshall J, Martin C, Pagliarello G, Tweeddale M, Schweitzer I, Yetisir E. A multicenter, randomized, controlled clinical trial of transfusion requirements in critical care. Transfusion Requirements in Critical Care Investigators, Canadian Critical Care Trials Group. N Engl J Med. 1999;340:409–17.
57. Netzer G, Liu X, Harris AD, Edelman BB, Hess JR, Shanholtz C, Murphy DJ, Terrin ML. Transfusion practice in the intensive care unit: a 10-year analysis. Transfusion. 2010;50:2125–34.
58. Murphy DJ, Needham DM, Netzer G, Zeger SL, Colantuoni E, Ness P, Pronovost PJ, Berenholtz SM. RBC transfusion practices among critically ill patients: has evidence changed practice? Crit Care Med. 2013;41:2344–53.
59. Hajjar LA, Vincent JL, Galas FR, Nakamura RE, Silva CM, Santos MH, Fukushima J, Kalil FR, Sierra DB, Lopes NH, Mauad T, Roquim AC, Sundin MR, Leao WC, Almeida JP, Pomerantzeff PM, Dallan LO, Jatene FB, Stolf NA, Auler Jr JO. Transfusion requirements after cardiac surgery: the TRACS randomized controlled trial. JAMA. 2010;304:1559–67.
60. Walsh TS, Boyd JA, Watson D, Hope D, Lewis S, Krishan A, Forbes JF, Ramsay P, Pearse R, Wallis C, Cairns C, Cole S, Wyncoll D. Restrictive versus liberal transfusion strategies for older mechanically ventilated critically ill patients: a randomized pilot trial. Crit Care Med. 2013;41:2354–63.
61. Naidech AM, Shaibani A, Garg RK, Duran IM, Liebling SM, Bassin SL, Bendok BR, Bernstein RA, Batjer HH, Alberts MJ. Prospective, randomized trial of higher goal hemoglobin after subarachnoid hemorrhage. Neurocrit Care. 2010;13:313–20.
62. Carson JL, Terrin ML, Noveck H, Sanders DW, Chaitman BR, Rhoads GG, Nemo G, Dragert K, Beaupre L, Hildebrand K, Macaulay W, Lewis C, Cook DR, Dobbin G, Zakriya KJ, Apple FS, Horney RA, Magaziner J. Liberal or restrictive transfusion in high-risk patients after hip surgery. N Engl J Med. 2011;365:2453–62.
63. Vincent JL. Transfusion triggers: getting it right! Crit Care Med. 2012;40:3308–9.
64. Vincent JL. Indications for blood transfusions: too complex to base on a single number? Ann Intern Med. 2012;157:71–2.
65. Holst LB, Haase N, Wetterslev J, Wernerman J, Aneman A, Guttormsen AB, Johansson PI, Karlsson S, Klemenzson G, Winding R, Nebrich L, Albeck C, Vang ML, Bulow HH, Elkjaer JM, Nielsen JS, Kirkegaard P, Nibro H, Lindhardt A, Strange D, Thormar K, Poulsen LM, Berezowicz P, Badstolokken PM, Strand K, Cronhjort M, Haunstrup E, Rian O, Oldner A, Bendtsen A, Iversen S, Langva JA, Johansen RB, Nielsen N, Pettila V, Reinikainen M, Keld D, Leivdal S, Breider JM, Tjader I, Reiter N, Gottrup U, White J, Wiis J, Andersen LH, Steensen M, Perner A. Transfusion requirements in septic shock (TRISS) trial – comparing the effects and safety of liberal versus restrictive red blood cell transfusion in septic shock patients in the ICU: protocol for a randomised controlled trial. Trials. 2013;14:150.

Parasuram Krishnamoorthy, Debabrata Mukherjee,
and Saurav Chatterjee

Abstract

There have been remarkable advancements in treating acute coronary syndrome with different angioplasty techniques, novel antithrombotic and antiplatelet agents, and heart failure therapies using mechanical assist devices. However, most of these interventions are done in patients with complex comorbidities, which lead to an increased risk of bleeding. Anemia is one of the most prevalent coexisting conditions in patients with heart failure and acute coronary syndrome. There is growing evidence that anemia in these patient populations is an independent predictor of mortality and adverse outcomes. Increasing the hemoglobin through blood transfusion should in theory increase oxygen delivery and reduce myocardial ischemia. However, there are several risks associated with transfusion. Randomized trials in some patient populations have demonstrated that restrictive use of blood transfusion, using a hemoglobin trigger of <7 g/dL, is associated with similar or even better outcomes compared with a liberal transfusion strategy using 10 g/dL as a transfusion trigger. However, it is not clear which strategy is safest for patients with ischemic heart disease or heart failure. The aim of this chapter is to describe and attempt to understand the pathophysiology of anemia in heart failure and ischemic heart disease and summarize recent advances and evidence behind using blood transfusion to treat anemia in patients with heart disease.

P. Krishnamoorthy, MD
Internal Medicine, Englewood Medical Center, New Jersey, NJ, USA

D. Mukherjee, MD
Division of Cardiology, Texas Tech University Health Sciences Center, El Paso, TX, USA

S. Chatterjee, MD (✉)
Division of Cardiology, St Luke's-Roosevelt Hospital Center,
Clark Building, 1111 Amsterdam Avenue, New York, NY, USA
e-mail: SChatterjee@chpnet.org

© Springer International Publishing Switzerland 2015
N.P. Juffermans, T.S. Walsh (eds.), *Transfusion in the Intensive Care Unit*,
DOI 10.1007/978-3-319-08735-1_4

4.1   Introduction

Advanced congestive heart failure (CHF) and coronary artery disease (CAD) are commonly associated with anemia. Approximately 4–61 % [1–16] of patients with CHF and 10–20 % [17–19] of patients with CAD have anemia. Variability in prevalence of anemia is attributable to varying and inconsistent definition of anemia reported in each study. There is ample evidence that anemia in heart disease is associated with adverse clinical outcomes like worsening of symptoms, decreased exercise tolerance and quality of life, as well as increased hospitalization and mortality rates [20–23].

Different strategies have been tried for treating anemia in patients with heart disease, including intravenous iron, erythropoiesis-stimulating agents, and red blood cell (RBC) transfusion. The aim of this chapter is to describe and understand the pathophysiology of anemia in heart diseases and to summarize recent advances and evidence of using RBC transfusion for treating anemia in patients with heart disease, including potential risks and benefits.

4.2   Cardiac Oxygen Consumption

The heart has the highest resting oxygen consumption per tissue mass compared to other organs in our body. The resting coronary blood flow is 250 ml/min, which represents approximately 5 % of cardiac output. Also oxygen extraction, defined as the difference between arterial and venous concentrations in oxygen (CaO_2–CvO_2), is high in the heart, with 70–80 % compared to 25 % for the rest of the body. In addition, there is an observed fivefold increase in the oxygen consumption during any exertion like exercise. Hence, increase in oxygen consumption must be met by an increase in coronary blood flow, which is impaired in the setting of anemia due to low oxygen content.

4.3   Pathophysiology of Anemia in Heart Disease

Deficiency in new erythrocyte production relative to the rate of removal of old erythrocytes causes anemia. Erythropoietin, a glycoprotein hormone produced primarily by the kidney, plays a pivotal role in tissue oxygen delivery and red blood cell homeostasis by preventing apoptosis of progenitor red blood cells [24, 25]. Any abnormality in renal production or decreased bone marrow response to erythropoietin can result in anemia.

Many factors probably contribute to the development of anemia in heart disease, including comorbid chronic kidney disease, blunted erythropoietin production, hemodilution, advanced age, aspirin-induced gastrointestinal blood loss, the use of renin–angiotensin–aldosterone system blockers, cytokine-mediated inflammation, gut malabsorption, and iron deficiency [16, 19]. Anemia is seen commonly in patients

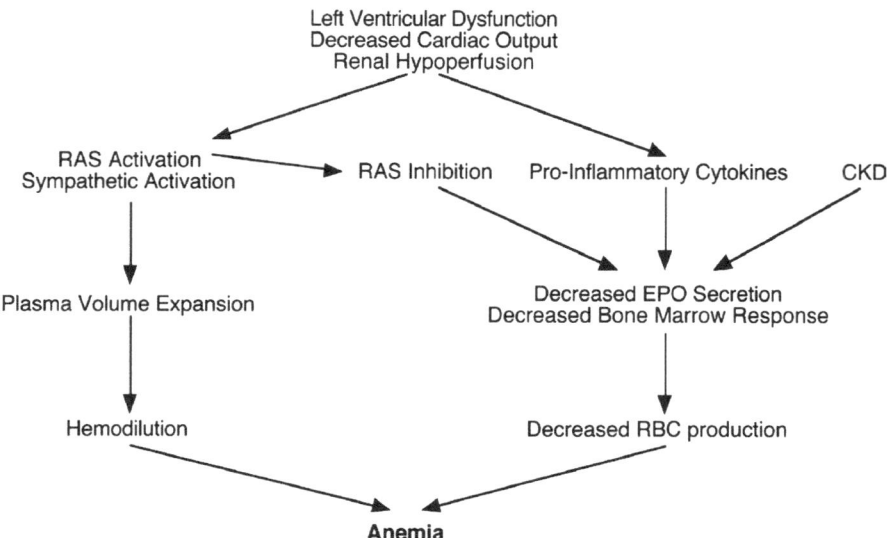

Fig. 4.1 Cardiorenal anemia syndrome in congestive heart failure (Tang and Katz [16])

with more severe symptoms (30–61 %) when compared with less symptomatic ambulatory populations (4–23 %) [16], but some reports indicate that anemia is also prevalent in patients with CHF and preserved ejection fraction [26–28]. Iron deficiency is reported only in <30 % of patients with heart disease, and hence most of the anemia is normocytic. Cardiorenal anemia syndrome is an important concept in CHF pathophysiology. This entity is a complex vicious cycle of congestive heart failure, chronic kidney disease, and anemia, each entity compounding the severity of the others via numerous mechanisms, some long understood, and others newly realized as explained in Fig. 4.1.

Anemia in CHF has multiple causes and effects. Ventricular dysfunction causes backward failure and venous congestion, producing hypervolemia with hemodilution, but also forward failure with hypoperfusion and ischemic damage to critical organs including the kidney. Advancing renal failure produces not only uremia and accelerated atherosclerosis but also decreases erythropoietin production and may be aggravated by angiotensin-converting enzyme inhibitors and angiotensin II receptor blockers. These drugs also may suppress erythropoiesis, thus aggravating similar effects of inflammatory cytokines, which are typically elevated in CHF. Uremia produces platelet dysfunction, which may aggravate aspirin-induced gastric bleeding. Bowel edema and the general debility of CHF lead to malnutrition and poor iron and vitamin absorption. This multifactorial anemia reduces capacity and, if severe enough, further stresses the compromised heart for which cardiac work is increased as part of the physiological response to anemia. It is at this arc of the vicious cycle that clinicians commonly believe that erythropoietin therapy or RBC transfusion may improve cardiac function and patient status.

4.4   Hemoglobin Triggers for Transfusion in Patients with Heart Disease

Patients with coexisting heart disease tolerate moderate normovolemic hemodilution or acute anemia well, provided that normovolemia is maintained [29–32]. However, an aggressive hemodilution, including normovolemic hemodilution, can cause myocardial ischemia that is reversible with a blood transfusion [33]. Among patients refusing any blood transfusions for religious reasons who have coexisting cardiovascular disease, postoperative hemoglobin levels below 6.0 g/dL were associated with an increased mortality and morbidity, and an increasingly greater difference in mortality and morbidity was observed between patients with and without coexisting cardiovascular diseases [34]. The question of when to transfuse an individual patient with a coexisting cardiac disease thus remains unanswered except at extremely low hemoglobin levels (e.g., <6.0 g/dL). Blood transfusions may be indicated in some anemic patients with coexisting cardiac disease [34–37].

Pooled data from randomized controlled trials in heterogeneous patient populations show that restricting blood transfusions to patients whose hemoglobin drops below 7 g/dL results in a significant reduction in total mortality, acute coronary syndrome, pulmonary edema, rebleeding, and bacterial infection, compared to a more liberal transfusion strategy [38]. The number needed to treat to save one life was 33. This strategy resulted in a 40 % reduction in the number of patients receiving a blood transfusion, with an average of 2 units less per person; however, over one-half of patients were still transfused.

Observational studies have consistently shown that transfusions are associated with an increased risk for adverse events after controlling for potential confounding variables, even when using a restrictive transfusion strategy [39–41]. It has been the traditional teaching that patients with cardiac ischemia should have a more liberal transfusion strategy to maintain oxygenation, but pooled observational studies show that transfusions are associated with especially high risk when given during an acute coronary syndrome [42, 43]. For patients with non-acute cardiac disease, subgroup analysis of data from a trial in critically ill patients showed that the restrictive strategy was not associated with worse outcomes for critically ill patients with cardiovascular disease [44].

It remains impossible to determine the optimum hemoglobin/hematocrit number at which a transfusion would be indicated generally and hence guidelines published in 2006 by the American Society of Anesthesiologists which state that "the decision of red blood cell transfusions should be based on the patient's risk of developing complications of inadequate oxygenation" is valid even for patients with coexisting cardiovascular disease [36]. It is therefore important to recognize signs of inadequate oxygenation in patients with coexisting heart diseases. Inadequate oxygenation may become manifest locally in the form of myocardial ischemia or globally in the form of a general hemodynamic instability with a tendency to hypotension and tachycardia despite normovolemia [33]. Myocardial ischemia may be detected by continuous electrocardiogram (ECG) monitoring and by transesophageal echocardiography. New ST-segment depressions of greater than 0.1 mV or new

Table 4.1 Transfusion indication in patients with coexisting cardiac diseases

	Evidence based/ scientific	Intraoperatively and ICU
New ST-segment depression >0.1 mV	Yes	Yes
New ST-segment elevation >0.2 mV	Yes	Yes
New wall motion abnormality in TEE	Yes	Yes
Oxygen extraction rate	>50 %	>40 %
SvO$_2$	<50 %	<60 %
Decrease in oxygen consumption	>10–50 %	>10 %
Hemoglobin transfusion triggers[a]		
All patients	6 g/dL	7 g/dL
Patients >80 years		7–8 g/dL
Patients with severe CAD		8 g/dL
Patients with signs of CHF		8 g/dL
Patients on >1 catecholamine infusion		8 g/dL
Patients with SaO$_2$ <90 %		8–9 g/dL

Abbreviations: *CAD* coronary artery disease, *CHF* congestive heart failure, *SvO$_2$* mixed venous oxygen saturation, *TEE* transesophageal echocardiography
[a]A blood transfusion is indicated at hemoglobin levels below the indicated threshold without specific sign of inadequate oxygenation. The listed parameters are only an indication for a blood transfusion after correction of hypovolemia, optimization of anesthesia, and ventilation and the correction of a tachycardia (if any). Blood transfusions, however, are not mandatory in each case

ST-segment elevations of greater than 0.2 mV for more than 1 min are generally regarded as a marker of myocardial ischemia (Table 4.1) [33]. During progressive hemodilution, one observes mostly ST-segment depression, suggesting subendocardial ischemia. In controlled studies such anemia-related ischemia is reversible by decreasing the heart rate, if elevated, and by minimal transfusion to increase the hemoglobin by 1–2 g/dL [45]. Also, new wall motion abnormalities clinically detected by transesophageal echocardiography are suggestive of myocardial ischemia and can be treated by an increase in the hemoglobin of only 1–2 g/dL.

Early signs of an inadequate circulation are a general hemodynamic instability characterized by a relative tachycardia and hypotension, an oxygen extraction rate of greater than 50 %, a low mixed-venous oxygen partial pressure (PvO$_2$), and a decrease in oxygen consumption [33]. In a position paper of the College of American Pathologists, an oxygen extraction rate of greater than 50 %, a PvO$_2$ less than 25 mmHg, and a reduction in oxygen consumption to less than 50 % of baseline are described as threshold values above which a blood transfusion would be indicated [35]. An oxygen extraction of greater than 50 % has been found to indicate exhaustion of compensatory mechanism in several studies and thus represents a clear transfusion indication [46, 47]. In contrast, a threshold of 25 mmHg for PvO$_2$ appears very low, since the PvO$_2$ decreases below the threshold of 25 mmHg only after circulatory collapse. A PvO$_2$ threshold of 32 mmHg appears more reasonable, because oxygen consumption started to decrease at a PvO$_2$ of 32 mmHg during progressive normovolemic hemodilution in pigs [33]. A decrease in oxygen consumption by greater than 50 % at normovolemia is certainly a transfusion indication; however, such a large reduction usually is observed only after hemodynamic collapse. Indeed, oxygen consumption decreases very late. Therefore, any decrease of greater than 10 % in oxygen consumption at low hemoglobin levels should be viewed as a potential sign of a compromised oxygenation of the organism, and a blood transfusion should be considered, provided that normovolemia has been achieved [48].

The main goal of blood transfusions is to increase oxygen-carrying capacity and mitigate myocardial ischemia, but experimental studies indicate no increase in tissue oxygenation and improvement in clinical outcomes with transfusion in any setting or with any nadir hemoglobin level [39, 49, 50]. This inability to improve oxygen uptake in vital organs is due to the hemodynamic response to increased blood viscosity as well as to chemical changes in red cells during preservation and storage, such as depletion of 2,3 diphosphoglycerate and nitric oxide, that diminish the ability of transfusion to deliver oxygen [51–55]. With millions of blood transfusions given yearly over the past century, it would be hard to calculate how many deaths may have been contributed to by transfusions. The adverse effects seen with blood transfusions, including bacterial infections, acute respiratory distress syndrome, multiorgan failure, rebleeding, and total mortality, may be due to an inflammatory response to the transfused blood product. Very little mechanistic explanation is known for no benefit or increased risk with transfusion using liberal strategy among patients with anemia and ACS. One such recent work by Silvain et al. found that blood transfusion was associated with modest but significant increase in measures of platelet reactivity and was more robust in patients previously on P2Y12 inhibitors [56]. At present, there is no randomized trial evidence that blood transfusions improve oxygen delivery or clinical outcomes in any setting, which underscores the urgent need for a randomized control trial of transfusion strategies especially in patients with ACS and CHF. There are two randomized trials, the CRIT study [57] and the MINT trial [58] examining liberal vs restrictive transfusion strategy in patients with ACS and had contrasting results. However, they had small sample sizes and were grossly underpowered to make any relevant conclusions regarding clinically important intervention effects and essentially showed divergent results on clinical outcomes such as mortality.

There remains an urgent and unmet need, as noted in recent guidelines [59], for more studies to help guide clinicians in finding optimal treatment threshold and options in the setting of anemia and bleeding in patients with ACS and CHF.

4.5   Conclusions

With the limited available evidence, we conclude that a restrictive transfusion strategy with a hemoglobin transfusion trigger of <7 g/dL might be safely practiced in patients with ischemic heart disease, including stable coronary artery disease and acute coronary syndrome unless they are symptomatic from anemia. We believe that at this threshold, benefits of transfusion probably exceed the risks. For patients who are symptomatic even at rest, hemoglobin transfusion trigger for these patients could be <8 g/dL. Also, other individual factors like severity of myocardial ischemia, plans for coronary artery revascularization, and rate of blood loss should be considered. Our conclusions are similar to European practice guidelines published recently where transfusion is recommended for hemoglobin of less than 8 g/dL or symptomatic from anemia in patients with unstable angina or non-ST-segment elevation MI [59].

References

1. Silverberg DS, Wexler D, Blum M, Keren G, Sheps D, Leibovitch E, Brosh D, Laniado S, Schwartz D, Yachnin T, Shapira I, Gavish D, Baruch R, Koifman B, Kaplan C, Steinbruch S, Iaina A. The use of subcutaneous erythropoietin and intravenous iron for the treatment of the anemia of severe, resistant congestive heart failure improves cardiac and renal function and functional cardiac class, and markedly reduces hospitalizations. J Am Coll Cardiol. 2000;35:1737–44.
2. Al-Ahmad A, Rand WM, Manjunath G, Konstam MA, Salem DN, Levey AS, Sarnak MJ. Reduced kidney function and anemia as risk factors for mortality in patients with left ventricular dysfunction. J Am Coll Cardiol. 2001;38:955–62.
3. Androne AS, Katz SD, Lund L, LaManca J, Hudaihed A, Hryniewicz K, Mancini DM. Hemodilution is common in patients with advanced heart failure. Circulation. 2003;107:226–9.
4. Ezekowitz JA, McAlister FA, Armstrong PW. Anemia is common in heart failure and is associated with poor outcomes: insights from a cohort of 12 065 patients with new-onset heart failure. Circulation. 2003;107:223–5.
5. Mozaffarian D, Nye R, Levy WC. Anemia predicts mortality in severe heart failure: the prospective randomized amlodipine survival evaluation (PRAISE). J Am Coll Cardiol. 2003;41:1933–9.
6. Horwich TB, Fonarow GC, Hamilton MA, MacLellan WR, Borenstein J. Anemia is associated with worse symptoms, greater impairment in functional capacity and a significant increase in mortality in patients with advanced heart failure. J Am Coll Cardiol. 2002;39:1780–6.
7. Cromie N, Lee C, Struthers AD. Anaemia in chronic heart failure: what is its frequency in the UK and its underlying causes? Heart. 2002;87:377–8.
8. Kosiborod M, Smith GL, Radford MJ, Foody JM, Krumholz HM. The prognostic importance of anemia in patients with heart failure. Am J Med. 2003;114:112–9.
9. McClellan WM, Flanders WD, Langston RD, Jurkovitz C, Presley R. Anemia and renal insufficiency are independent risk factors for death among patients with congestive heart failure admitted to community hospitals: a population-based study. J Am Soc Nephrol. 2002;13:1928–36.
10. Tanner H, Moschovitis G, Kuster GM, Hullin R, Pfiiffner D, Hess OM, Mohacsi P. The prevalence of anemia in chronic heart failure. Int J Cardiol. 2002;86:115–21.
11. Felker GM, Gattis WA, Leimberger JD, Adams KF, Cuffe MS, Gheorghiade M, O'Connor CM. Usefulness of anemia as a predictor of death and rehospitalization in patients with decompensated heart failure. Am J Cardiol. 2003;92:625–8.
12. Anand IS, Kuskowski MA, Rector TS, Florea VG, Glazer RD, Hester A, Chiang YT, Aknay N, Maggioni AP, Opasich C, Latini R, Cohn JN. Anemia and change in hemoglobin over time related to mortality and morbidity in patients with chronic heart failure: results from Val-HeFT. Circulation. 2005;112:1121–7.
13. Szachniewicz J, Petruk-Kowalczyk J, Majda J, Kaczmarek A, Reczuch K, Kalra PR, Piepoli MF, Anker SD, Banasiak W, Ponikowski P. Anaemia is an independent predictor of poor outcome in patients with chronic heart failure. Int J Cardiol. 2003;90:303–8.
14. Wexler D, Silverberg D, Sheps D, Blum M, Keren G, Iaina A, Schwartz D. Prevalence of anemia in patients admitted to hospital with a primary diagnosis of congestive heart failure. Int J Cardiol. 2004;96:79–87.

15. Maggioni AP, Opasich C, Anand I, Barlera S, Carbonieri E, Gonzini L, Tavazzi L, Latini R, Cohn J. Anemia in patients with heart failure: prevalence and prognostic role in a controlled trial and in clinical practice. J Card Fail. 2005;11:91–8.
16. Tang YD, Katz SD. Anemia in chronic heart failure: prevalence, etiology, clinical correlates, and treatment options. Circulation. 2006;113:2454–61.
17. Malyszko J, Bachorzewska-Gajewska H, Malyszko J, Levin-Iaina N, Iaina A, Dobrzycki S. Prevalence of chronic kidney disease and anemia in patients with coronary artery disease with normal serum creatinine undergoing percutaneous coronary interventions: relation to New York Heart Association class. Isr Med Assoc J. 2010;12:489–93.
18. Boyd CM, Leff B, Wolff JL, Yu Q, Zhou J, Rand C, et al. Informing clinical practice guideline development and implementation: prevalence of coexisting conditions among adults with coronary heart disease. J Am Geriatr Soc. 2011;59:797–805.
19. Kansagara D, Dyer E, Englander H, Freeman M, Kagen D. Treatment of anemia in patients with heart disease: a systematic review. Ann Intern Med. 2013;159(11):746–57.
20. O'Meara E, Clayton T, McEntegart MB, McMurray JJ, Lang CC, Roger SD, et al. CHARM Committees and Investigators. Clinical correlates and consequences of anemia in a broad spectrum of patients with heart failure: results of the Candesartan in Heart Failure: Assessment of Reduction in Mortality and Morbidity (CHARM) Program. Circulation. 2006;113:986–94.
21. Komajda M, Anker SD, Charlesworth A, Okonko D, Metra M, Di Lenarda A, et al. The impact of new onset anaemia on morbidity and mortality in chronic heart failure: results from COMET. Eur Heart J. 2006;27:1440–6.
22. da Silveira AD, Ribeiro RA, Rossini AP, Stella SF, Ritta HA, Stein R, et al. Association of anemia with clinical outcomes in stable coronary artery disease. Coron Artery Dis. 2008;19:21–6.
23. Sabatine MS, Morrow DA, Giugliano RP, Burton PB, Murphy SA, McCabe CH, et al. Association of hemoglobin levels with clinical outcomes in acute coronary syndromes. Circulation. 2005;111:2042–9.
24. Katz SD. Mechanisms and treatment of anemia in chronic heart failure. Congest Heart Fail. 2004;10:243–7.
25. Bauer C, Kurtz A. Oxygen sensing in the kidney and its relation to erythropoietin production. Annu Rev Physiol. 1989;51:845–56.
26. Berry C, Hogg K, Norrie J, Stevenson K, Brett M, McMurray J. Heart failure with preserved left ventricular systolic function: a hospital cohort study. Heart. 2005;91:907–13.
27. Brucks S, Little WC, Chao T, Rideman RL, Upadhya B, Wesley-Farrington D, Sane DC. Relation of anemia to diastolic heart failure and the effect on outcome. Am J Cardiol. 2004;93:1055–7.
28. Klapholz M, Maurer M, Lowe AM, Messineo F, Meisner JS, Mitchell J, Kalman J, Phillips RA, Steingart R, Brown Jr EJ, Berkowitz R, Moskowitz R, Soni A, Mancini D, Bijou R, Sehhat K, Varshneya N, Kukin M, Katz SD, Sleeper LA, Le Jemtel TH. Hospitalization for heart failure in the presence of a normal left ventricular ejection fraction: results of the New York Heart Failure Registry. J Am Coll Cardiol. 2004;43:1432–8.
29. Spahn DR, Schmid ER, Seifert B, Pasch T. Hemodilution tolerance in patients with coronary artery disease who are receiving chronic beta-adrenergic blocker therapy. Anesth Analg. 1996;82:687–94.
30. Spahn DR, Casutt M. Eliminating blood transfusions: new aspects and perspectives. Anesthesiology. 2000;93:242–55.
31. Herregods L, Foubert L, Moerman A, Francois K, Rolly G. Comparative study of limited intentional normovolaemic haemodilution in patients with left main coronary artery stenosis. Anaesthesia. 1995;50:950–3.
32. Spahn DR, Seifert B, Pasch T, Schmid ER. Effects of chronic beta-blockade on compensatory mechanisms during isovolaemic haemodilution in patients with coronary artery disease. Br J Anaesth. 1997;78:381–5.
33. Spahn DR, Dettori N, Kocian R, Chassot PG. Transfusion in the cardiac patient. Crit Care Clin. 2004;20(2):269–79.
34. Carson JL, Noveck H, Berlin JA, Gould SA. Mortality and morbidity in patients with very low postoperative Hb levels who decline blood transfusion. Transfusion. 2002;42:812–8.

35. Simon TL, Alverson DC, AuBuchon J, Cooper ES, DeChristopher PJ, Glenn GC, et al. Practice parameter for the use of red blood cell transfusions: developed by the Red Blood Cell Administration Practice Guideline Development Task Force of the College of American Pathologists. Arch Pathol Lab Med. 1998;122:130–8.
36. Nuttall GA, Brost BC, Connis RT, Gessner JS, Harrison CR, Miller RD, et al. American Society of Anesthesiologists Task Force on Perioperative Blood Transfusion and Adjuvant Therapies. Anesthesiology. Practice guidelines for perioperative blood transfusion and adjuvant therapies: an updated report by the American Society of Anesthesiologists Task Force on Perioperative Blood Transfusion and Adjuvant Therapies. Anesthesiology. 2006;105(1):198–208.
37. Ferraris VA, Ferraris SP, Saha SP, et al. Perioperative blood transfusion and blood conservation in cardiac surgery: the Society of Thoracic Surgeons and The Society of Cardiovascular Anesthesiologists clinical practice guideline. Ann Thorac Surg. 2007;83(5 Suppl):S27–86.
38. Salpeter SR, Buckley JS, Chatterjee S. Impact of more restrictive blood transfusion strategies on clinical outcomes: a meta-analysis and systematic review. Am J Med. 2013. doi:10.1016/j.amjmed.2013.09.017. pii: S0002-9343(13)00841-3.
39. Tinmouth A, Fergusson D, Yee IC, Hebert PC. Clinical consequences of red cell storage in the critically ill. Transfusion. 2006;46(11):2014–27.
40. Reeves BC, Murphy GJ. Increased mortality, morbidity, and cost associated with red blood cell transfusion after cardiac surgery. Curr Opin Cardiol. 2008;23(6):607–12.
41. Hill GE, Frawley WH, Griffith KE, Forestner JE, Minei JP. Allogeneic blood transfusion increases the risk of postoperative bacterial infection: a meta-analysis. J Trauma. 2003;54(5):908–14.
42. Rao SV, Jollis JG, Harrington RA, et al. Relationship of blood transfusion and clinical outcomes in patients with acute coronary syndromes. JAMA. 2004;292(13):1555–62.
43. Chatterjee S, Wetterslev J, Sharma A, Lichstein E, Mukherjee D. Association of blood transfusion with increased mortality in myocardial infarction: a meta-analysis and diversity-adjusted study sequential analysis. Arch Intern Med. 2012;24:1–8.
44. Hebert PC, Yetisir E, Martin C, et al. Is a low transfusion threshold safe in critically ill patients with cardiovascular diseases? Crit Care Med. 2001;29(2):227–34.
45. Spahn DR, Smith RL, Veronee CD, McRae RL, Hu W, Menius AJ, et al. Acute isovolemic hemodilution and blood transfusion: effects on regional function and metabolism in myocardium with compromised coronary blood flow. J Thorac Cardiovasc Surg. 1993;105:694–704.
46. Spahn DR, Leone BJ, Reves JG, Pasch T. Cardiovascular and coronary physiology of acute isovolemic hemodilution: a review of nonoxygen-carrying and oxygen-carrying solutions. Anesth Analg. 1994;78:1000–21.
47. Wilkerson DK, Rosen AL, Gould SA, Sehgal LR, Sehgal HL, Moss GS. Oxygen extraction ratio: a valid indicator of myocardial metabolism in anemia. J Surg Res. 1987;42:629–34.
48. Spahn DR, Schanz U, Pasch T. Perioperative transfusionskriterien. Anaesthesist. 1998;47:1011–20.
49. Hebert PC, McDonald BJ, Tinmouth A. Clinical consequences of anemia and red cell transfusion in the critically ill. Crit Care Clin. 2004;20(2):225–35.
50. Napolitano LM, Corwin HL. Efficacy of red blood cell transfusion in the critically ill. Crit Care Clin. 2004;20(2):255–68.
51. Marik PE, Sibbald WJ. Effect of stored-blood transfusion on oxygen delivery in patients with sepsis. JAMA. 1993;269(23):3024–9.
52. Berezina TL, Zaets SB, Morgan C, et al. Influence of storage on red blood cell rheological properties. J Surg Res. 2002;102(1):6–12.
53. McMahon TJ, Ahearn GS, Moya MP, et al. A nitric oxide processing defect of red blood cells created by hypoxia: deficiency of S-nitrosohemoglobin in pulmonary hypertension. Proc Natl Acad Sci U S A. 2005;102(41):14801–6.
54. Bennett-Guerrero E, Veldman TH, Doctor A, et al. Evolution of adverse changes in stored RBCs. Proc Natl Acad Sci U S A. 2007;104(43):17063–8.
55. Reynolds JD, Ahearn GS, Angelo M, Zhang J, Cobb F, Stamler JS. S-nitrosohemoglobin deficiency: a mechanism for loss of physiological activity in banked blood. Proc Natl Acad Sci U S A. 2007;104(43):17058–62.

56. Silvain J, Abtan J, Kerneis M, Martin R, Finzi J, Vignalou JB, Barthelemy O, O'Connor SA, Luyt CE, Brechot N, Mercadier A, Brugier D, Galier S, Collet JP, Chastre J, Montalescot G. Impact of red blood cell transfusion on platelet aggregation and inflammatory response in anemic coronary and non-coronary patients the TRANSFUSION-2 study. J Am CollCardiol. 2014;63(13):1289–96.
57. Aronson D, Dann EJ, Bonstein L, et al. Impact of red blood cell transfusion on clinical outcomes in patients with acute myocardial infarction. Am J Cardiol. 2008;102(2):115–9.
58. Carson JL, Brooks MM, Abbott JD, Chaitman B, Kelsey SF, Triulzi DJ, Srinivas V, Menegus MA, Marroquin OC, Rao SV, Noveck H, Passano E, Hardison RM, Smitherman T, Vagaonescu T, Wimmer NJ, Williams DO. Liberal versus restrictive transfusion thresholds for patients with symptomatic coronary artery disease. Am Heart J. 2013;165(6):964–971.e1.
59. Carson JL, Grossman BJ, Kleinman S, Tinmouth AT, Marques MB, Fung MK, Holcomb JB, Illoh O, Kaplan LJ, Katz LM, Rao SV, Roback JD, Shander A, Tobian AA, Weinstein R, Swinton McLaughlin LG, Djulbegovic B, Clinical Transfusion Medicine Committee of the AABB. Red blood cell transfusion: a clinical practice guideline from the AABB*. Ann Intern Med. 2012;157(1):49.

Red Blood Cell Transfusion Trigger in Cardiac Surgery

Gavin J. Murphy, Nishith N. Patel,
and Jonathan A.C. Sterne

Abstract

In cardiac surgery, the principal aim of red blood cell transfusion is to maintain oxygen delivery and prevent tissue hypoxia in the setting of acute anaemia and severe bleeding. Both these clinical indications are common, and over 50 % of all cardiac surgery patients receive red blood cell transfusion, utilising a significant proportion of blood service resources in developed countries. Severe anaemia accounts for the vast majority of all red blood cells used; however, there is uncertainty as to what constitutes a safe level of anaemia or a trigger for transfusion. There is also uncertainty as to the risks and benefits of transfusion; experimental and early clinical studies suggest that transfusion may promote organ injury. Existing blood management guidelines recommend restrictive transfusion practice, and this is supported by observational analyses in cardiac surgery patients showing strong associations between transfusion and adverse outcome. However, these studies fail to address the important clinical question as to what constitutes the anaemia threshold where transfusion is indicated. They are also beset my multiple sources of bias that confound analysis and contribute to

G.J. Murphy (✉)
Department of Cardiovascular Sciences, University of Leicester, Clinical Sciences Wing,
Glenfield General Hospital, Leicester LE3 9QP, UK
e-mail: gjm19@le.ac.uk

N.N. Patel
Academic Cardiac Surgery Group, National Heart and Lung Institute,
Imperial College London, Hammersmith Hospital,
DuCane Road, London W12 0NN, UK
e-mail: nishith.patel@imperial.ac.uk

J.A.C. Sterne
School of Social and Community Medicine, University of Bristol,
Canynge Hall, 39 Whatley Road, Bristol BS8 2PS, UK
e-mail: jonathan.sterne@bristol.ac.uk

© Springer International Publishing Switzerland 2015
N.P. Juffermans, T.S. Walsh (eds.), *Transfusion in the Intensive Care Unit*,
DOI 10.1007/978-3-319-08735-1_5

inflated estimates of risk. RCTs in non-cardiac surgery patients do not demonstrate harm from more restrictive thresholds (lower haematocrits) and suggest that this is the best practice. These studies do not reflect the lack of cardiovascular reserve in cardiac surgery patients, however, that is often compounded by the abnormal oxygen utilisation that follows cardiopulmonary bypass. Meta-analyses of RCTs in cardiac surgery appear to support a benefit for more liberal thresholds. These analyses are dominated however by a single large study, the Transfusion Indication Threshold Reduction (TITRe 2) trial, that demonstrated a benefit from a more liberal transfusion threshold of 9 g/dL. We conclude therefore that in the absence of high-quality evidence to the contrary, cardiac surgery patients may be considered a specific high-risk group where restrictive transfusion practice will promote harm.

5.1   Introduction

The aim of perioperative red blood cell (RBC) transfusion in cardiac surgery is to improve or preserve oxygen delivery in the setting of blood loss and anaemia, with the intention of preventing oxygen supply dependency and organ injury. Cardiac surgery is characterised by a high prevalence of anaemia. Perioperative anaemia, defined arbitrarily as a haemoglobin concentration <12 g/dL, is common, affecting over 75 % of patients [1, 2]. It occurs as a consequence of low preoperative red blood cell mass; haemodilution during surgery, including the use of crystalloid prime; perioperative blood loss; and decreased haematopoiesis as a consequence of chronic disease or as a result of a perioperative inflammatory state [1, 2]. Red blood cell transfusion is the preferred and most rapid treatment for acute anaemia in this setting. Cardiac surgery is also characterised by a high prevalence of coagulopathy and severe bleeding [3, 4]. Red blood cell transfusion in the setting of severe blood loss and incipient haemorrhagic shock is clearly lifesaving. Studies in trauma indicate that massive red blood cell transfusion in isolation may not adequately treat bleeding patients however and suggest that these should be accompanied by high ratios of non-red blood cell to red blood cell components if best outcomes are to be achieved. This has not been demonstrated thus far in cardiac surgery. Red blood cell transfusion rates in clinical studies, typically in the range of 45–95 % [5, 6], far outstrip estimates of coagulopathic or severe bleeding, estimated in up to 15 % of patients, depending on the definition used [3, 7]. Although it has not been clearly demonstrated, this suggests that the greater proportion of all red blood cells transfused are for the treatment of anaemia.

5.1.1   Consequences of Anaemia During Cardiac Surgery

Anaemia is associated with an increased risk of developing low cardiac output, acute kidney injury, and death in cardiac surgery [1, 2, 8, 9]. However, there is uncertainty as to the anaemia threshold below which tissues develop hypoxia and injury. Observational studies have demonstrated increased neurological and renal injury once haematocrits fall below 24 % [8, 9]. Oxygen supply and utilisation are different in cardiac surgery as compared to other patient groups. This is because these patients often demonstrate impaired autoregulation and tissue hypoxia during cardiopulmonary bypass (CPB) that is attributed to non-pulsatile blood flow in the setting of microvascular dysfunction, as commonly observed in patients with diabetes, hypertension and those with severe peripheral vascular disease. Cardiac surgery patients also commonly demonstrate oxygen supply dependency postoperatively despite apparently adequate oxygen delivery [10], probably due in part to systemic inflammation and mitochondrial dysfunction that occurs as a consequence of CPB. It should also be remembered that cardiac surgery patients at the outset are at the limits of their cardiovascular reserve; the principal indication for cardiac surgery is *symptomatic* cardiac disease [11, 12]. Safe levels of anaemia may therefore change with time and be patient specific, and higher levels of haemoglobin may be required to prevent oxygen supply dependency in this population. This raises the question as to whether it is possible to define a universal anaemia threshold below which tissue hypoxia is likely or, as is reflected in contemporary transfusion guidelines, a patient-specific threshold is required [13, 14].

5.1.2   Consequences of Red Blood Cell Transfusion in Cardiac Surgery

There is also uncertainty as to the potential harms from red blood cell transfusion. Experimental studies have demonstrated that red blood cell transfusion promotes lung, myocardial, and renal inflammation by the activation of platelet and leuco-cytes [15, 16]. This has been attributed to the 'storage lesion' whereby the accumulation of harmful and pro-inflammatory substances in the storage supernatant and deterioration in erythrocyte structure and function are thought to result in posttransfusion inflammation and organ injury in recipients [16]. Clinical studies support these observations; Koch and colleagues in a study of 6,001 patients at the Cleveland Clinic demonstrated that transfusion of older blood, stored for >14 days, was associated with an increase in pulmonary, renal, and cardiac complications compared to transfusion of blood stored for <14 days [17]. In a randomised cross-over trial, Weiskopf and colleagues demonstrated that transfusion of older red blood cells to healthy recipients resulted in altered lung function, although in these subjects, there was only a very modest effect of transfusion on conventional inflammatory markers [18].

5.1.3   Practice of Red Blood Cell Transfusion in Cardiac Surgery

Uncertainty as to the risks and benefits of anaemia and red blood cell transfusion is reflected by wide variations in red blood cell transfusion rates, ranging from 25 to 75 % between cardiac centres in the UK [5] and 8–93 % in the USA [6]. This variation represents a potentially modifiable source of morbidity and perhaps mortality. Variation in practice also has significant resource issues; cardiac surgery utilises 5 % of all red blood cells in the UK [19] and up to 25 % in the USA [20]. Incipient blood shortages, due to the effects of demographic shifts on the supply and demand of blood, mandate more appropriate use of this precious resource [21]. Variation in clinical practice arises due to the lack of high-quality evidence. Systematic reviews of the available evidence have increasingly advocated more restrictive practice; i.e. the toleration of lower levels of anaemia and less frequent transfusion [22]. Restrictive practice is also increasingly reflected in contemporary blood management guidelines [13, 14] as well as in health policy [23, 24]. Here we consider the strengths and limitations of the available evidence that is used to guide transfusion decisions in cardiac surgery.

5.2 Observational Studies on Red Blood Cell Transfusion in Cardiac Surgery

Observational studies uniformly demonstrate strong associations between red blood cell transfusion and low cardiac output, acute kidney injury, pulmonary injury, sepsis, increased use of healthcare resources, and death (Fig. 5.1 and associated references). The principal limitation of these studies is that they do not attempt to establish a safe level of anaemia below which transfusion may be beneficial, i.e. the

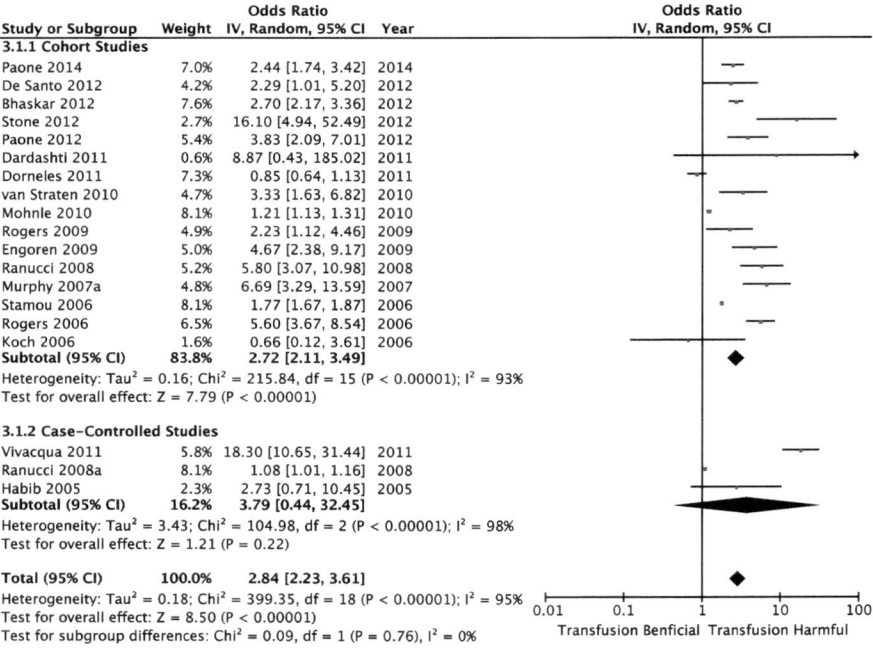

Fig. 5.1 Forest plot of the odds of mortality for transfusion versus no transfusion from observational studies. Individual references are available on request

principal clinical question they seek to address. Rather these trials compare transfusion with no transfusion. It follows that the estimated effects of transfusion from these studies are likely to have been subject to unmeasured confounding, because they included in the transfusion group patients who became so severely ill during surgery that they could never have remained transfusion-free. For example, almost none of these studies attempted to adjust for bleeding and the severity of perioperative anaemia, the two principal indications for red blood cell transfusion, which are also risk factors for adverse outcome. This also leads to lead time bias; these studies do not attempt to adjust for adverse events that are likely to have preceded transfusion. This is compounded when transfusion is considered as a categorical variable, as is the case in many of these studies. This assumes homogeneity in the transfused population. It is reasonable to suggest however that patients who receive massive transfusions will have a poor outcome due in part to other possibly unmeasured variables that precede transfusion, but by grouping these patients with those receiving single-unit transfusions, the estimates of the association between transfusion and adverse outcomes are both confounded and inflated. Studies that have attempted to consider the effects of anaemia, as distinct from transfusion, suffer from similar limitations. Overall, the observational studies published thus far lack the methodological rigour required to demonstrate a causal association between either anaemia or transfusion and adverse outcome. More importantly, they offer little evidence to support transfusion decisions in the setting of anaemia. This is best demonstrated by randomised controlled trials (RCTs).

5.3   Randomised Controlled Trials on Red Blood Cell Transfusion in Non-Cardiac Surgery Patients

A recent Cochrane review summarised the results of published RCTs that have attempted to determine safe levels of anaemia or appropriate transfusion threshold across a range of clinical settings [25]. These RCTs, commonly referred to as 'trigger trials', determine whether patient allocation to a more liberal transfusion threshold, based usually on a higher blood haematocrit or haemoglobin concentration, results in a different clinical outcome to a more restrictive or lower transfusion threshold. Thus, both groups are exposed to transfusion albeit at different frequencies and also to different levels of anaemia. In this respect, they differ from observational studies in that they do not attempt to define the risks of transfusion or anaemia in isolation and reflect the absolute interdependence of these two factors. This is pragmatic, there is no ethical basis upon which transfusion could be completely withheld from one group of patients, and they reflect the almost universal use of haemoglobin/haematocrit measurements to guide red blood cell transfusion decisions. These trials are limited in that they assume a universal anaemia threshold that is applicable to all patients and cannot inform individual treatment decisions, although this is commonplace in clinical practice and a criticism of all RCTs. Many of these trials also have design limitations that significantly increase the risk of bias. Firstly, most are underpowered to detect differences in important clinical endpoints such as

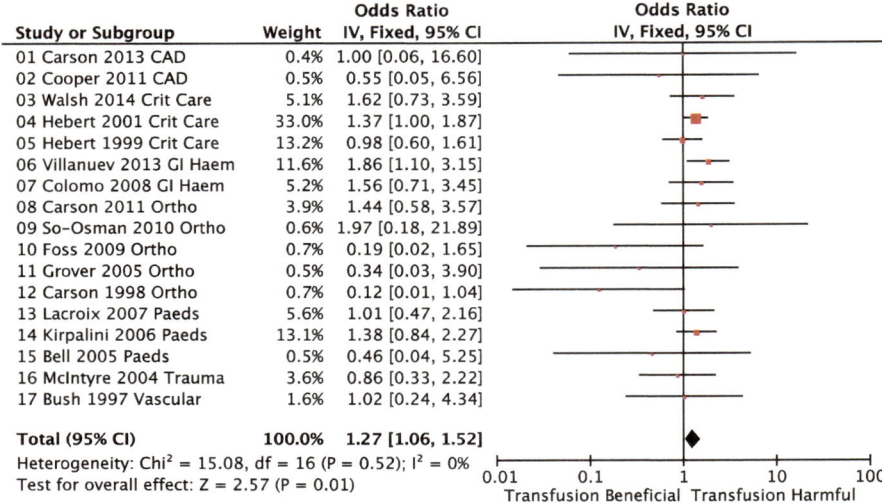

| | | Odds Ratio | Odds Ratio |
Study or Subgroup	Weight	IV, Fixed, 95% CI	IV, Fixed, 95% CI
01 Carson 2013 CAD	0.4%	1.00 [0.06, 16.60]	
02 Cooper 2011 CAD	0.5%	0.55 [0.05, 6.56]	
03 Walsh 2014 Crit Care	5.1%	1.62 [0.73, 3.59]	
04 Hebert 2001 Crit Care	33.0%	1.37 [1.00, 1.87]	
05 Hebert 1999 Crit Care	13.2%	0.98 [0.60, 1.61]	
06 Villanuev 2013 GI Haem	11.6%	1.86 [1.10, 3.15]	
07 Colomo 2008 GI Haem	5.2%	1.56 [0.71, 3.45]	
08 Carson 2011 Ortho	3.9%	1.44 [0.58, 3.57]	
09 So–Osman 2010 Ortho	0.6%	1.97 [0.18, 21.89]	
10 Foss 2009 Ortho	0.7%	0.19 [0.02, 1.65]	
11 Grover 2005 Ortho	0.5%	0.34 [0.03, 3.90]	
12 Carson 1998 Ortho	0.7%	0.12 [0.01, 1.04]	
13 Lacroix 2007 Paeds	5.6%	1.01 [0.47, 2.16]	
14 Kirpalini 2006 Paeds	13.1%	1.38 [0.84, 2.27]	
15 Bell 2005 Paeds	0.5%	0.46 [0.04, 5.25]	
16 McIntyre 2004 Trauma	3.6%	0.86 [0.33, 2.22]	
17 Bush 1997 Vascular	1.6%	1.02 [0.24, 4.34]	
Total (95% CI)	**100.0%**	**1.27 [1.06, 1.52]**	

Heterogeneity: Chi² = 15.08, df = 16 (P = 0.52); I² = 0%
Test for overall effect: Z = 2.57 (P = 0.01)

0.01   0.1   1   10   100
Transfusion Beneficial Transfusion Harmful

Fig. 5.2 Forest plot of the odds of mortality for restrictive transfusion versus liberal transfusion from non-cardiac surgery RCTs. Individual studies are as labelled in reference [25]

death. Secondly, randomised trials commonly recruit selected groups of relatively low-risk patients who have low frequencies of the adverse outcomes the intervention is intended to influence. Thirdly, by randomising all consented patients, many of whom never develop severe anaemia, they result in large proportions of patients in either group who never require transfusion. Finally, few of these studies report compliance to allocated transfusion thresholds, a potential source of procedural bias. These sources of bias tend to move the effect estimate of the intervention towards the null. Quantitative meta-analyses of the outcomes from these trials do not overcome all of these limitations. They are also limited in that they assume that the patient groups will be homogeneous, with a similar balance of risks and benefits over a wide range of restrictive and liberal transfusion thresholds in different clinical settings. Perhaps unsurprisingly, these meta-analyses show no apparent difference between restrictive and liberal transfusion strategies (Fig. 5.2). That is not to say that these findings must be discounted. They are supported by the findings of a recent large high-quality RCT in high-risk patients. The Functional Outcomes in Cardiovascular Patients Undergoing Surgical Hip Fracture Repair (FOCUS) trial compared liberal and restrictive transfusion thresholds in 2016 hip fracture patients, of whom 63 % had a history of cardiovascular disease. This trial only randomised patients with haemoglobin levels <10 g/dL and carefully documented non-adherence to the study protocol (8 %). The FOCUS trial reported no difference in a range of clinical outcomes, including death or major morbidity. Thus, best evidence suggests that restrictive transfusion is not harmful in non-cardiac surgery patients. Moreover, in the absence of harm, restrictive practice should be adopted; there is no clinical indication to provide a therapy that has no benefit but a considerable cost, as concluded by the Cochrane review [22, 25]. Importantly however, the patients in the

FOCUS and other trials did not have symptomatic cardiac disease and did not undergo surgery with cardiopulmonary bypass. Transfusion decisions in cardiac surgery are best informed by trials conducted in cardiac surgery patients.

5.4 Randomised Trials on Red Blood Cell Transfusion in Cardiac Surgery Patients

Six RCTs [26–31] have thus far compared liberal with restrictive transfusion practices in patients undergoing cardiac surgery in a total of 3,356 patients (Fig. 5.3). These trials demonstrate many of the limitations observed in non-cardiac surgery RCTs. In particular, all but 1 of these trials, the Transfusion Indication Threshold Reduction (TITRe 2) trial, did not select only those who required transfusion, i.e. those that developed predefined level of anaemia prior to randomisation. TITRe 2 was also the only trial adequately powered to demonstrate differences in important clinical outcomes. Meta-analysis of these trials is dominated by this and another trial, the single-centre Transfusion Requirements After Cardiac Surgery (TRACS) trial [20]. The TRACS trial randomised 502 patients to restrictive and liberal transfusion thresholds. However, all consented patients were randomised in this study, reducing the ability of the trial to detect a treatment effect; 22 % in the liberal group did not receive any transfusion despite a liberal trigger which was higher than in most other trials (haematocrit 30 %). In the TRACS trial, there was no difference between the groups with respect to death or major morbidity. The TITRe 2 trial was a multicentre trial in 16 UK cardiac centres that recruited 3,565 patients of whom 2007 breached the threshold of 9 g/dL and were randomised to either a restrictive threshold of 7.5 g/dL or a liberal threshold of 9 g/dL. Fifty-three percent of patients were transfused in the restrictive group, and 92 % were transfused in the liberal group. Non-adherence was closely monitored and was similar to that observed in the FOCUS trial (8 %). There was no difference between the two groups in terms of the primary outcome, a composite of any infectious or ischaemic complication. However, sensitivity analyses that included acute kidney

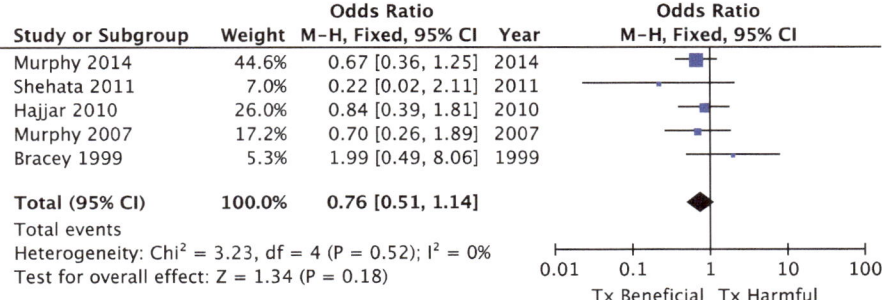

Fig. 5.3 Forest plot of the odds of mortality for restrictive transfusion versus liberal transfusion from cardiac surgery RCTs (Data extracted from references [26–31])

injury as objectively determined by serial creatinine measurements in the primary outcome did demonstrate increased risk of harm in the restrictive group (odds ratio for infectious or ischaemic morbidity = 1.20, 95 % confidence intervals (CI) 1.00–1.44, $p = 0.045$). This finding was supported by an analysis of secondary outcomes including death, which was increased in the restrictive group (4.2 % versus 2.6 %; hazard ratio = 1.64, 95 % CI 1.00–2.67, $p = 0.045$). Quantitative meta-analysis of all the trials that have compared liberal with restrictive transfusions in cardiac surgery also indicates a benefit from more liberal transfusion thresholds (Fig. 5.3), with, importantly, a reduced risk of death from liberal transfusion (OR = 0.76, 95 % CI 0.51–1.14). The cardiac surgery trials used different thresholds, and there is insufficient evidence from these trials to recommend a specific anaemia threshold. The TITRe 2 trial suggested that a threshold of 9 g/dL may be appropriate. Interestingly, subgroup analysis did not detect any interaction between the effect estimate and a range of risk factors including poor left ventricular function, diabetes, and age greater than 75 years, factors commonly used to influence transfusion decisions.

5.5   Summary and Conclusions

Contemporary blood management guidelines, and increasingly health policy, advocate restrictive transfusion practice, with the caveat that thresholds should be increased in high-risk patients. The use of restrictive thresholds is supported by the findings of observational studies and RCTs in non-cardiac surgery patients. These studies are not adequate to inform transfusion decisions in cardiac surgery however. Existing observational studies in cardiac surgery patients lack the methodological rigour to determine safe levels of anaemia, and the findings of RCTs in non-cardiac surgery patients fail to address the specific nature of the patients presenting for cardiac surgery, principally the existence of symptomatic disease, and the altered oxygen utilisation characteristic of CPB. RCTs in cardiac surgery have until recently suffered from significant limitations making interpretation difficult. However, the recent TITRe 2 trial, which has randomised significantly more patients than all the previous cardiac surgery RCTs combined, indicates that restrictive transfusion practice may not be safe in this highly specific clinical setting, and this is supported by quantitative meta-analysis of this and other cardiac surgery 'trigger' trials. Moreover, other risk factors that are often considered to influence transfusion requirements such as age and co-morbidity did not influence this result, further supporting a hypothesis that these patients exist at the limits of the oxygen supply/utilisation balance. Here we suggest that cardiac surgery therefore represents a specific high-risk group where restrictive practice is not safe. This hypothesis will be tested by the Transfusion Requirements in Cardiac Surgery III (TRACS III) trial (NCT02042898). TRACS III is an international multicentre RCT comparing liberal with restrictive thresholds that started recruiting in January 2014. This trial will enrol 3,592 patients, more than all previous trials combined that is powered to detect differences in death and major morbidity. However, until the results of this trial are presented, expected in 2018, the available evidence suggests that more liberal transfusion thresholds of a haemoglobin of 9 g/dL be adopted in cardiac surgery.

References

1. Karkouti K, Wijeysundera DN, Beattie WS. Risk associated with preoperative anemia in cardiac surgery: a multicenter cohort study. Circulation. 2008;117:478–84.
2. Kulier A, Levin J, Moser R, Rumpold-Seitlinger G, Tudor IC, Snyder-Ramos SA, Moehnle P, Mangano DT, Investigators of the Multicenter Study of Perioperative Ischemia Research Group; Ischemia Research and Education Foundation. Impact of preoperative anemia on outcome in patients undergoing coronary artery bypass graft surgery. Circulation. 2007; 116:471–9.
3. Unsworth-White MJ, Herriot A, Valencia O, Poloniecki J, Smith EE, Murday AJ, Parker DJ, Treasure T. Resternotomy for bleeding after cardiac operation: a marker for increased morbidity and mortality. Ann Thorac Surg. 1995;59:664–7.
4. Moulton MJ, Creswell LL, Mackey ME, Cox JL, Rosenbloom M. Reexploration for bleeding is a risk factor for adverse outcomes after cardiac operations. J Thorac Cardiovasc Surg. 1996;111:1037–46.
5. Bennett-Guerrero E, Zhao Y, O'Brien SM, Ferguson Jr TB, Peterson ED, Gammie JS, Song HK. Variation in use of blood transfusion in coronary artery bypass graft surgery. JAMA. 2010;304(14):1568–75.
6. Murphy MF, Murphy GJ, Gill R, Herbertson M, Allard S, Grant-Casey J. 2011 audit of blood transfusion in adult cardiac surgery. NHS Blood & Transplant. Available from: http://hospital.blood.co.uk/library/pdf/2011_Use_of_Blood_in_Adult_Cardiac_Surgery_report.pdf. Accessed 25 Aug 2014.
7. Karkouti K, Wijeysundera DN, Yau TM, Beattie WS, Abdelnaem E, McCluskey SA, Ghannam M, Yeo E, Djaiani G, Karski J. The independent association of massive blood loss with mortality in cardiac surgery. Transfusion. 2004;44:1453–62.
8. Ranucci M, Conti D, Castelvecchio S, Menicanti L, Frigiola A, Ballotta A, Pelissero G. Hematocrit on cardiopulmonary bypass and outcome after coronary surgery in nontransfused patients. Ann Thorac Surg. 2010;89:11–7.
9. Habib RH, Zacharias A, Schwann TA, Riordan CJ, Engoren M, Durham SJ, et al. Role of hemodilutional anemia and transfusion during cardiopulmonary bypass in renal injury after coronary revascularization: implications on operative outcome. Crit Care Med. 2005; 33:1749–56.
10. Utoh J, Moriyama S, Okamoto K, Kunitomo R, Hara M, Kitamura N. The effects of cardiopulmonary bypass on postoperative oxygen metabolism. Surg Today. 1999;29:28–33.
11. Task Force on Myocardial Revascularization of the European Society of Cardiology (ESC) and the European Association for Cardio-Thoracic Surgery (EACTS); European Association for Percutaneous Cardiovascular Interventions (EAPCI), Wijns W, Kolh P, Danchin N, et al. Guidelines on myocardial revascularization. Eur Heart J. 2010;31(20):2501–55.
12. Joint Task Force on the Management of Valvular Heart Disease of the European Society of Cardiology (ESC), European Association for Cardio-Thoracic Surgery (EACTS), Vahanian A, Alfieri O, Andreotti F, et al. Guidelines on the management of valvular heart disease (version 2012). Eur Heart J. 2012;33(19):2451–96.
13. Ferraris VA, Brown JR, Despotis GJ, et al. 2011 update to the Society of Thoracic Surgeons and the Society of Cardiovascular Anesthesiologists blood conservation clinical practice guidelines. Ann Thorac Surg. 2011;91(3):944–82.
14. Carson JL, Grossman BJ, Kleinman S, Tinmouth AT, Marques MB, Fung MK, Holcomb JB, Illoh O, Kaplan LJ, Katz LM, Rao SV, Roback JD, Shander A, Tobian AA, Weinstein R, Swinton McLaughlin LG, Djulbegovic B, Clinical Transfusion Medicine Committee of the AABB. Red blood cell transfusion: a clinical practice guideline from the AABB*. Ann Intern Med. 2012;157(1):49–58.
15. Patel NN, Lin H, Jones C, Walkden G, Ray P, Sleeman PA, Angelini GD, Murphy GJ. Interactions of cardiopulmonary bypass and erythrocyte transfusion in the pathogenesis of pulmonary dysfunction in swine. Anesthesiology. 2013;119:365–78.
16. Tinmouth A, et al. Clinical consequences of red cell storage in the critically ill. Transfusion. 2006;46(11):2014–27.

17. Koch CG, Li L, Sessler DI, Figueroa P, Hoeltge GA, Mihaljevic T, Blackstone EH. Duration of red-cell storage and complications after cardiac surgery. N Engl J Med. 2008; 358:1229–39.
18. Weiskopf RB, Feiner J, Toy P, Twiford J, Shimabukuro D, Lieberman J, Looney MR, Lowell CA, Gropper MA. Fresh and stored red blood cell transfusion equivalently induce subclinical pulmonary gas exchange deficit in normal humans. Anesth Analg. 2012;114(3):511–9.
19. Wells AW, Llewelyn CA, Casbard A, Johnson AJ, Amin M, Ballard S, Buck J, Malfroy M, Murphy MF, Williamson LM. The EASTER Study: indications for transfusion and estimates of transfusion recipient numbers in hospitals supplied by the National Blood Service. Transfus Med. 2009;19(6):315–28.
20. US Department of Health and Human Services. The 2007 nationwide blood collection and utilization survey report. Washington, DC: Dept of Health and Human Services; 2007.
21. Greinacher A, Fendrich K, Brzenska R, Kiefel V, Hoffmann W. Implications of demographics on future blood supply: a population-based cross-sectional study. Transfusion. 2011; 51(4):702–9.
22. Carson JL, Carless PA, Hébert PC. Outcomes using lower vs higher hemoglobin thresholds for red blood cell transfusion. JAMA. 2013;309(1):83–4.
23. Farmer SL, Towler SC, Leahy MF, Hofmann A. Drivers for change: Western Australia Patient Blood Management Program (WA PBMP), World Health Assembly (WHA) and Advisory Committee on Blood Safety and Availability (ACBSA). Best Pract Res Clin Anaesthesiol. 2013;27(1):43–58.
24. World Health Organization. Global forum for blood safety: patient blood management: priorities for action. Dubai; 2011. Available from: URL: http://www.who.int/bloodsafety/events/gfbs_01_pbm/en/index.html. Cited 20 Jul 2013.
25. Carson JL, Carless PA, Hebert PC. Transfusion thresholds and other strategies for guiding allogeneic red blood cell transfusion. Cochrane Database Syst Rev. 2012;4:CD002042.
26. Shehata N, Burns LA, Nathan H, et al. A randomized controlled pilot study of adherence to transfusion strategies in cardiac surgery. Transfusion. 2012;52(1):91–9.
27. Murphy GJ, Rizvi SI, Battaglia F, et al. A pilot randomized controlled trial of the effect of transfusion- threshold reduction on transfusion rates and morbidity after cardiac surgery. Transfus Altern Transfus Med. 2007;9 Suppl 1:41–2.
28. Slight RD, Fung AK, Alonzi C, Bappu NJ, McClelland DB, Mankad PS. Rationalizing blood transfusion in cardiac surgery: preliminary findings with a red cell volume-based model. Vox Sang. 2007;92(2):154–6.
29. Bracey AW, Radovancevic R, Riggs SA, et al. Lowering the hemoglobin threshold for transfusion in coronary artery bypass procedures: effect on patient outcome. Transfusion. 1999;39(10):1070–7.
30. Hajjar LA, Vincent JL, Galas FR, et al. Transfusion requirements after cardiac surgery: the TRACS randomized controlled trial. JAMA. 2010;304(14):1559–67.
31. Brierley R, et al. A multi-centre randomised controlled trial of Transfusion Indication Threshold Reduction on transfusion rates, morbidity and healthcare resource use following cardiac surgery: Study protocol. Transfus Apher Sci. 2014;50(3):451–61.

Red Blood Cell Transfusion Trigger in Brain Injury

6

Shane W. English, Dean Fergusson, and Lauralyn McIntyre

Abstract

The neurocritically ill patient population is a unique patient group whose disease processes are a common reason for intensive care unit (ICU) admission. Brain injury patients are typically younger than general ICU patients, and the significant morbidity and mortality associated with them makes their potential life years lost enormous. The overriding goal in management is the prevention of secondary neurologic injury. It is biologically plausible that correction of low hemoglobin with red blood cell (RBC) transfusion may improve outcomes through an increase in oxygen delivery. This study question has not been adequately tested, and these patients have not been well represented in the existing quality trials that provide the key evidence that guides red blood cell (RBC) transfusion in many other critically ill populations. In this chapter, we review the physiologic and clinical significance of anemia as well as the evidence for RBC transfusion in three important neurocritically ill patient subgroups: those with ischemic stroke, traumatic brain injury, and intracranial hemorrhage (intracerebral hemorrhage and subarachnoid hemorrhage).

S.W. English (✉) • L. McIntyre
Centre for Transfusion Research, Clinical Epidemiology Program,
Ottawa Hospital Research Institute, Ottawa, ON, Canada

Department of Medicine (Critical Care), The University of Ottawa,
The Ottawa Hospital, Ottawa, ON, Canada
e-mail: senglish@ohri.ca

D. Fergusson
Centre for Transfusion Research, Clinical Epidemiology Program,
Ottawa Hospital Research Institute, Ottawa, ON, Canada

© Springer International Publishing Switzerland 2015
N.P. Juffermans, T.S. Walsh (eds.), *Transfusion in the Intensive Care Unit*,
DOI 10.1007/978-3-319-08735-1_6

6.1 Oxygen Transport and Anemia Physiology in the Normal Brain

The brain relies on the steady delivery of oxygenated arterial blood to maintain normal function. The oxygen content of arterial blood (C_aO_2) is determined predominantly by hemoglobin concentration ([Hb]) and oxygen saturation (S_aO_2) and to a very small extent by partial pressure of oxygen in arterial blood (P_aO_2):

$$C_aO_2 = [Hb] \times S_aO_2 + 0.0031 \times P_aO_2.$$

Oxygen delivery (DO_2) is in turn dependent not only on oxygen content but, as expressed by the equation $DO_2 = CO \times C_aO_2$, is also dependent upon cardiac output (CO)[1]. DO_2 to the brain is dependent on cerebral blood flow (CBF). CBF determinants include brain compliance, blood viscosity, and vascular resistance.

Although hemoglobin concentration is directly related to DO_2, the hematocrit, which is a contributor to blood viscosity, is inversely related to CBF. Normal brain oxygen delivery is approximately 150 ml O_2/min, which is approximately triple of what the brain consumes (VO_2) under normal conditions [2]. An increase in VO_2 or a decrease in any DO_2 variable requires a compensatory change to maintain adequate oxygen delivery as well as the ability to compensate for hypoxia and ischemic insult. Normal brain responses to a decrease in hemoglobin (anemia), which decreases C_aO_2, include increases in heart rate, stoke volume (to increase CO), and a decrease in blood viscosity to improve cerebral blood flow [3]. In brain injury, CBF determinants such as brain compliance, blood viscosity, and vascular resistance may be altered. In addition, the normal compensatory mechanisms to anemia may be disrupted.

6.2 Oxygen Transport and Anemia Physiology in the Injured Brain

Following brain injury, many processes can result in secondary injury including alterations in cerebral metabolism, ischemia, tissue hypoxia, or the downstream effects of these processes [4]. A decrease in arterial oxygen content and/or a change in CBF are central, potentially reversible causes of secondary injury. Contributing factors can include anemia, hypoxemia, elevated intracranial pressure, vasospasm, loss or compromised cerebral autoregulation, and uncoupling of flow and metabolism [5]. Vasospasm plays a particularly important role following subarachnoid hemorrhage, but all of these processes can be present to varying degrees in all etiologies of brain injury.

Patients suffering from acute neurological stresses including ischemic stroke, traumatic brain injury, and intracranial hemorrhage are thought to be particularly susceptible to secondary ischemia from altered or decreased tissue oxygen delivery and/or tissue oxygen uptake and utilization. The normal physiologic vasodilation in response to anemia (and decreased C_aO_2) leads to increased cerebral blood volume and may potentiate hyperemia, edema, and increased intracranial pressure.

As physiologic compensatory responses to anemia are exhausted or stretched, secondary ischemic injury may occur, which can further worsen a vicious cycle of edema, increased pressure, and altered cerebral blood flow. The net result is propagation of the ischemic injury.

Numerous preclinical models of brain injury exist which have improved the understanding of the pathophysiology of anemia in brain injury. In a rat model of traumatic brain injury, anemia was shown to increase hypoxic cerebral injury after neurotrauma compared to otherwise healthy controls [6]. In a mathematical modeling exercise using a rabbit model of stroke, a hemoglobin of 10 g/dL was the anemia threshold below which oxygen uptake in the ischemic penumbra decreased [7]. These animal models suggest that the injured brain may be susceptible to anemia.

Following brain injury in humans, anemia appears to exacerbate tissue hypoxia. In a prospective evaluation of 20 consecutive patients with severe subarachnoid hemorrhage (Hunt and Hess 4 or 5), Oddo et al. [8] demonstrated that a hemoglobin of <9 g/dL was associated with lower brain tissue oxygen levels and increased levels of lactate and pyruvate, which are metabolic markers of cellular hypoxia; these were consistent with greater brain hypoxia. This association remained significant after adjustment for other important variables in the subarachnoid hemorrhage patient population (cerebral perfusion pressure, central venous pressure, vasospasm, and P_aO_2/F_iO_2 ratio). In another small study of eight subarachnoid hemorrhage patients with vasospasm, isovolemic hemodilution was shown to increase cerebral blood flow but decrease global cerebral delivery rate of oxygen [9]. Both cerebral blood flow and oxygen delivery were decreased in hypervolemic hemodilution, and an increase in ischemic brain volume was seen at a hematocrit of 0.28 (approximately 8 g/dL).

In summary, there is a strong pathophysiological rationale, and some supportive clinical data, that the injured brain is more susceptible to the effects of anemia than other organs. This may be potentiated when normal compensatory mechanisms are exhausted or altered, making the acute brain-injured population a unique and potentially distinct subgroup from other critical care populations with respect to anemia and its management.

6.3 Epidemiology and Clinical Impact of Anemia in Brain Injury

Anemia in the critically ill is common, with up to 70 % of patients suffering some degree of hemoglobin (Hb) drop and 30 % having a Hb < 10 g/dL at some point over the course of their ICU stay [10–12]. The brain injury patient is also at high risk for anemia. Several recent reviews have summarized the existing data on anemia and its management in brain injury [3, 5, 13, 14]. A hemoglobin of <12 g/dL in females and <13 g/dL in males was observed in 97 % of severe ischemic stroke patients (defined as an ICU length of stay >5 days) in a recent small single-center cohort study [15]. Anemia in severe traumatic brain injury, defined as a post-resuscitation Glasgow Coma Scale score of 8 or less, is common and affects up to 50 % of these patients [3]. Similarly, moderate anemia (Hb < 10 g/dL) in aneurysmal subarachnoid hemorrhage, which is the most common type of primary subarachnoid hemorrhage, affects more than 50 % of cases [14, 16]. In this group, anemia develops within a mean of 3.5 days (median = 2 days) from admission and is associated with female sex, history of hypertension, poor clinical grade of subarachnoid hemorrhage, and a baseline hematocrit <36 % [16].

The etiology of anemia in neurocritical care patients is multifactorial and thereby mimics that of other ICU populations. Causes include blood loss (i.e., both disease related and iatrogenically driven from procedures and frequent phlebotomy) as well as inflammatory-related consumption, myelosuppression, and erythropoietin and iron metabolism abnormalities [15, 16].

In brain injury, both anemia that is prevalent at baseline and anemia that develops following the neurologic event appear to be associated with adverse clinical outcomes [3]. The vast majority of the evidence, however, is retrospective in nature and subject to the many limitations inherent to these types of study. It is not entirely clear whether anemia is purely a marker of comorbid illness and disease severity or if it is independently a poor prognostic factor.

6.3.1 Impact of Anemia in Ischemic Stroke

In a study of 135 consecutive ischemic stroke patients, the relationship between baseline hemoglobin and infarct size at presentation as well as between baseline hemoglobin and infarct progression was examined [17]. The authors determined that baseline hemoglobin was inversely related to both initial infarct size and infarct progression, which remained significant when controlling for age, gender, admission glucose, time to diagnosis, and stroke subtype. Decreasing hemoglobin levels also predicted poor functional outcome and mortality after ischemic stroke at 3 months [18]. The same authors more recently demonstrated that among severe ischemic stroke patients (admitted for >5 days to ICU), lower hemoglobin and anemia (hemoglobin <12 g/dL in women and <13 g/dL in men) were independently associated with longer ICU length of stay and duration of mechanical ventilation. However, anemia was not associated with mortality or adverse long-term outcome in their sample [15]. The authors attribute the lack of an association between anemia and mortality to two important limitations: (1) their retrospective study was limited to a severely injured patient population whose severe neurologic injuries may have predefined these outcomes, and (2) the study may not have been sufficiently powered to detect a signal of effect.

6.3.2 Impact of Anemia in Traumatic Brain Injury

Anemia has been demonstrated to be negatively associated with TBI outcome in several studies. Whether present at baseline or developing during the acute stages of illness, anemia appears to be associated with increased mortality and poor functional outcome. A recent single-center retrospective cohort study of 169 ICU patients with severe TBI demonstrated that 7-day mean hemoglobin of <9 g/dL was associated with an increase of more than three times the odds of hospital mortality than those with a mean hemoglobin ≥9 g/dL, after controlling for age, Glasgow Coma Scale scores, ventricular drain insertion, and RBC transfusion [19]. A subsequent narrative review identified 14 observational studies examining the association of anemia with outcome, of which more than half demonstrated a negative association between anemia and outcome [20]. This association may be particularly important in patients with evidence of brain tissue hypoxia [21]. However, the limitations of observational data are illustrated by a retrospective study in 169 severe TBI patients, which found an association between anemia and death or poor neurologic outcome, which disappeared when correcting for disease severity and other known predictors of poor outcome. In this study, an increase in duration of time spent with a hematocrit <30 % was associated with improved outcome [22]. The authors speculated that this finding might be explained by a subgroup of patients with low hemoglobin that had not undergone RBC transfusion, suggesting that RBC transfusion had adverse effects. These findings highlight the significant limitation of confounding by indication in observational studies.

6.3.3 Impact of Anemia in Intracranial Hemorrhage

In a recent observational study of 435 consecutive patients with primary intracerebral hemorrhage [23], anemia at admission (defined as Hb < 12 g/dL in men and <13 g/dL in women) was associated with larger hemorrhage volumes and higher probability of mortality at 1 year and was an independent predictor of poor functional outcome at 1 year. This contradicted earlier retrospective studies that demonstrated that nadir or mean hemoglobin, not admission hemoglobin, was associated with poor functional status at hospital discharge but not mortality [24, 25].

In subarachnoid hemorrhage, anemia is independently associated with poor outcome (adjusted for age, hemorrhage grade, aneurysm size, rebleed, and cerebral infarction from vasospasm) [26, 27], regardless of the severity of the subarachnoid hemorrhage [28]. In the absence of RBC transfusion, higher mean hemoglobin levels have been associated with a decreased risk of death or hospital discharge to nursing home or skilled nursing facility [29]. Whether better outcomes can be achieved with RBC transfusion remains unknown.

In summary, in the neurocritical care population, anemia appears to negatively impact outcome across a variety of patient subgroups. These data are however predominantly from retrospective observational studies and are limited due to confounding. Despite a strong physiologic rationale for RBC transfusion, it is unclear whether clinical outcomes are positively impacted by treatment of anemia with transfusion.

6.4   Effects of RBC Transfusion in the Injured Brain

Preclinical studies have demonstrated the biologic plausibility of oxygen delivery optimization in brain injury. Investigations using recent techniques for monitoring brain tissue oxygen demonstrate the benefit of improved oxygen delivery to tissue at risk from ischemia [4, 8]. Oxygen delivery (DO_2) is improved with RBC transfusion as a result of increased hemoglobin concentration. For instance, observational work in brain-injured adults found that brain tissue partial pressure of oxygen is higher with higher hemoglobin concentrations [8] and, in most patients, increases with red blood cell transfusion [30]. In a prospective observational study of 35 consecutive patients with brain injury, RBC transfusion resulted in a mean increase in brain tissue oxygen by 49 %, unrelated to changes in cerebral perfusion pressure [30]. Moreover, measurement of oxygen delivery in human brains with vasospasm following subarachnoid hemorrhage demonstrated no increase with induced hypertension or fluid bolus but did significantly improve with RBC transfusion in patients with anemia (hemoglobin <9 g/dL) [31]. Perhaps equally as important, the resultant increase in hemoglobin post transfusion did not translate into a drop in CBF as a consequence of the increased viscosity. A small study of eight subarachnoid hemorrhage patients with anemia (hemoglobin <10 g/dL) demonstrated stable cerebral blood flow, an increase in oxygen delivery, and a decrease in oxygen extraction fraction following an RBC transfusion [32]. Finally, another small study of 17 subarachnoid hemorrhage patients with vasospasm, published by the same authors as an abstract [33], demonstrated that cerebral oxygen delivery improved post transfusion when targets were <10 g/dL. Transfusion above this level was associated with a drop in cerebral blood flow.

Given that hemoglobin concentration is directly related to oxygen delivery, the above findings are not surprising. However, improved delivery does not guarantee increased oxygen uptake or utilization nor improved clinical outcomes. In the non-neurologic critically ill population, it is clear that RBC transfusion increases DO_2, but this has not always translated into a similar positive impact on oxygen consumption (VO_2) [34–38]. Even in states of anemia, RBC transfusion in the critically ill has not consistently demonstrated an increase in VO_2 [39, 40]. Older studies have showed that septic patients with a pre-transfusion low oxygen extraction fraction [36] or without a lactic acidosis [41] have an increase in VO_2 following RBC transfusion, which may suggest a benefit. Understanding whether clinical outcomes change as a result of RBC transfusion to increase oxygen delivery following brain injury is essential, because pathophysiologic outcomes may not translate into clinical benefit. The decision to transfuse must always balance the potential benefits of increased oxygen delivery with the inherent risks of RBC transfusion.

6.5   Observational and Randomized Controlled Intervention Studies of the Clinical Effects of RBC Transfusion in the Injured Brain

Observational data in human subjects with various brain injury etiologies have demonstrated conflicting effects of RBC transfusion on the outcome. Although several randomized trials have examined the potential benefit of a restrictive versus liberal transfusion strategy in the management of critically ill patients, the few neurocritically ill patients in these studies significantly limit their generalizability to this patient population.

The most robust randomized comparison of a restrictive versus a liberal transfusion strategy in a mixed critically ill population is the TRICC trial [42]. Among general ICU patients, those transfused at a restrictive hemoglobin trigger of 7 g/dL had no difference in outcome as compared to patients transfused at a liberal hemoglobin trigger of 10 g/dL and actually trended toward a lower 28-day mortality (18.7 versus 23.3 %, $p=0.11$) with less organ dysfunction and cardiac complications. However, few patients with neurologic injury were included in this study.

A recent systematic review of comparative studies of RBC transfusion in the neurocritically ill published prior to 2011 [43] found only six relevant citations in the literature. All were at high risk of bias, and there was a lack of long-term outcome assessment in the included papers. Of the six citations, four were in TBI patients, one in subarachnoid hemorrhage, and one in a mixed population. These will be reviewed in the subsections below, but overall, no benefit in mortality or lengths of hospital stay was demonstrated in the lower transfusion trigger groups. The authors concluded that insufficient evidence exists to support or refute a restrictive transfusion trigger in the neurocritical care population.

6.5.1   RBC Transfusion Trigger in Ischemic Stroke

Following ischemic stroke, like other areas of brain injury, maintaining euvolemia is extremely important as is optimizing oxygen delivery to "at-risk" hypoperfused areas around the infarcted brain (penumbra) to prevent infarct extension. The 2013 AHA Guidelines for the Early Management of Ischemic Stroke [44] provides no guidance with regard to the role of RBC transfusion to treat anemia and/or optimize oxygen delivery. An elevated hematocrit and resultant increased blood viscosity have been shown to contribute to hypoperfusion, increased infarct size, and increased mortality [3]. However, hemodilution or volume expansion in the acute phases has failed to lead to a reduction in mortality or functional dependence. Despite initially promising results of using high-dose albumin in the early hours of stroke management, a large phase III clinical trial was stopped early due to futility [45]. Additionally, more pulmonary edema was seen in the intervention arm. A number of studies examining the optimal hematocrit level in ischemic stroke patients point to a level of 0.40–0.45 [5]. The only study that has looked at the impact of RBC transfusion in ischemic stroke is the single-center retrospective cohort study by

Kellert et al. published in 2014 [15]. In their cohort of severe ischemic stroke patients (required ICU admission for ≥5 days), the 32 % of patients that received RBC transfusion(s) were more likely to undergo tracheostomy and other interventions and had longer ICU lengths of stay and duration on mechanical ventilation. No correlation was found between RBC transfusion and either in-hospital mortality or 3-month neurologic outcome; however, a regression model was not performed to control for important potential confounders. Further, this study is likely underpowered and limited to ICU patients.

6.5.2 RBC Transfusion Trigger in Traumatic Brain Injury

Like other areas of neurocritical care, there is a lack of evidence to guide RBC transfusion in traumatic brain injury patients. The Brain Trauma Foundation Guidelines [46], now widely disseminated and adopted into clinical practice, make no specific recommendation to guide this aspect of care.

In the small subgroup analysis of the neurologic patients ($n = 67$) in the TRICC trial [47], the authors could not demonstrate harm in the restrictive transfusion strategy group but were also unable to demonstrate benefit in the liberal transfusion group. These patients had all suffered from trauma or isolated closed-head injuries as adjudicated by the primary research team. The very small sample makes this difficult to interpret but suggests that a restrictive transfusion strategy may well be safe. A small retrospective study that examined the effect of a hemoglobin ≥9.8 g/dL following the early resuscitative and operative phase of severe TBI failed to demonstrate any benefit or harm, regardless of whether RBC transfusion was required to achieve this level [48]. Two other retrospective studies included in the previously mentioned systematic review [43] that compared patients who received at least one RBC transfusion when their hemoglobin was between 7 and 10 g/dL as compared to those who did not receive transfusion and also did not demonstrate a mortality difference [49, 50]. The non-transfused patients tended to have shorter ICU and hospital lengths of stay. In these studies, it is impossible to disentangle transfusion effect from the effect of different severities of anemia. Similar results are reported from a small pediatric subgroup analysis of a previously published RCT. In this analysis, two transfusion thresholds were compared; however, only 3 of the 66 patients experienced the outcome (mortality) [51]. No randomized controlled trial comparing a liberal to a restrictive RBC transfusion strategy or optimal transfusion trigger has ever been completed.

Too little evidence exists to draw evidence-based guidelines on optimal hemoglobin targets or transfusion trigger in TBI. Based on evidence of poor outcomes with low hemoglobin in populations at risk of cerebral ischemia and physiologic data supporting RBC transfusion, but a lack of clear benefit from a liberal RBC transfusion strategy, the British Committee for Standards in Haematology makes the following recommendations [5]:

1. In patients with TBI, the target hemoglobin should be 7–9 g/dL.
2. In patients with TBI and evidence of cerebral ischemia, the target hemoglobin should be >9 g/dL.

6.5.3 RBC Transfusion Trigger in Intracranial Hemorrhage

Similar to other management guidelines in neurocritical care, the 2010 American Heart Association "Guidelines for the Management of Spontaneous Intracerebral Hemorrhage" [52] makes no recommendation regarding the treatment of anemia or the utility of RBC transfusion in intracranial hemorrhage patients. Evidence guiding RBC transfusion in this population is scant and derived solely from observational data. These data have led to conflicting findings regarding RBC transfusion and outcome. For example, Chang et al. [24] found in their single-center retrospective study of 109 patients that RBC transfusion was associated with a nine times greater odds ratio of poor neurologic recovery or death in a univariate analysis. Of note, when other factors including age, intracranial hemorrhage severity, nadir hemoglobin, and the need for intubation were controlled for in multivariable regression analysis, statistical significance was lost, though a signal remained. Diedler et al. [25] found in their retrospective cohort of 247 patients that RBC transfusion was not associated with poor neurologic outcome or mortality in either univariate or multivariate analysis. However, in this study, only those patients with a hemoglobin of 10 g/dL or less were reviewed for possible RBC transfusion accounting for an RBC transfusion rate of only 5 %.

The majority of the existing data on RBC transfusion in subarachnoid hemorrhage are derived from observational studies. In a study of 421 patients with subarachnoid hemorrhage, Levine et al. demonstrated that the use of RBC transfusion was associated with an increased risk of infection including pneumonia and septicemia as well as prolonged mechanical ventilation (8.7 vs 6.1 days, $p=0.007$) [53]. Two studies [28, 54] suggested that the administration of RBC transfusions were associated with poor neurological outcome and that this relationship may be stronger among patients who do not suffer from vasospasm [27]. However, after adjusting for disease severity and age, this association was no longer significant ($p=0.08$, OR not reported) [29]. In contrast, two observational studies published in 2009 and 2012 did not detect associations between RBC transfusions and ICU mortality and long-term functional or neurological outcomes [55, 56].

All of these observational studies in SAH have significant limitations. As in other observational studies, these include potential selection bias, confounding due to indication, and residual confounding. Like the aforementioned studies, they are all single centered and include limited or no baseline adjustments or no time-dependent adjustments for confounding influences. Also, most studies preceded 2005. With the publication of the influential ISAT study [57] which provoked a major shift from surgical clipping to interventional coiling of ruptured aneurysms, management of subarachnoid hemorrhage patients has changed since 2005. Coiling is associated with less mortality, less neurologic disability, and fewer technical complications as compared to clipping [57, 58]. The impact of this significant management change on the incidence and management of anemia in subarachnoid hemorrhage is unclear.

A post hoc analysis of two small RCTs (studying statin and erythropoietin therapy in subarachnoid hemorrhage, respectively), which included 160 patients, demonstrated in a multivariate analysis that RBC transfusion was associated with poor outcome as measured with the Glasgow Outcome Scale (GOS) [59]. The only RBC transfusion threshold randomized controlled trial in an adult brain injury patient population is in subarachnoid hemorrhage patients. This small randomized trial of 44 patients compared a lower (10 g/dL) versus a higher (11.5 g/dL) hemoglobin transfusion threshold strategy with outcomes of safety and 14- and 28-day independent functional outcomes [60]. The authors demonstrated a comparable safety profile but no significant difference with respect to 28-day functional status. With the primary aim to demonstrate safety, this trial was not powered to determine the effect of different transfusion thresholds on meaningful clinical outcomes. Also of note, the thresholds selected for this trial were higher than currently stated practice thresholds [61]. Current stated RBC transfusion practice in subarachnoid hemorrhage patients among intensivists and neurosurgeons surveyed in North America suggests that most observe a restrictive transfusion strategy in low-grade disease but are more liberal and more likely to transfuse in high-grade disease, in the presence of vasospasm or delayed cerebral ischemia, or with documented low brain tissue oxygen tension.

The most recent American Heart Association Guidelines for the Management of Aneurysmal SAH contains the new recommendation to consider RBC transfusion in SAH patients at risk for cerebral ischemia [58]. The threshold of when to transfuse or to what target hemoglobin is not known nor recommended in the AHA guidelines. The evidence guiding anemia management and RBC transfusion triggers is limited at best and predominantly observational in nature with a significant lack of randomized controlled trials with meaningful clinical outcomes. Stating these same limitations, the British Committee for Standards in Haematology recommends a target hemoglobin of 8–9 g/dL for patients with subarachnoid hemorrhage [5].

6.6   Ongoing Studies

There are ongoing small neurocritical care studies which are examining the role of RBC transfusion in brain injury management:

- Effect of Red Blood Cell Transfusion on Brain Metabolism in Patients with Subarachnoid Hemorrhage (NCT00968227): Washington University School of Medicine study planning 48 patient enrollment to determine the change in proportion of brain regions with low oxygen delivery pre- and post-RBC transfusion (primary outcome) and the relationship between change in oxygen delivery and angiographic vasospasm (secondary outcome)
- Study of Cerebral Tissue Oxygenation During Transfusion in Traumatic Brain Injury (NIRS TBI) (NCT01728831): Canadian-led prospective observation study of 30 patients examining the ability of a near-infrared spectroscopy to provide noninvasive objective measure of physiologic effect of RBC transfusion

Although these studies have the potential to make significant contributions related to understanding physiology and surrogate outcomes, they are not adequate to examine clinical outcomes. There are no ongoing/registered trials (http://www.clinicaltrials.gov) examining the effect of RBC transfusion on the outcome in the neurocritical care population. These studies are urgently needed.

6.7 Summary

Limited, mostly single-center retrospective observations suggest that anemia negatively impacts outcome in the brain-injured patient. Preclinical and clinical physiologic data support the utility of RBC transfusion in brain injury. However, there is little clinical evidence to guide RBC transfusion in brain injury patients. There are no randomized controlled trials in adult neurocritical care populations powered for clinically meaningful outcomes to guide management. Although the existing observational data seem to suggest that transfusion may in fact negatively impact outcome (similar to other critical care populations), these studies are limited due to confounding. It is crucial to complete randomized controlled trials of RBC transfusion strategies in these patients because their morbidity and mortality is great and there is strong physiologic rationale to transfuse.

Current evidence supports a restrictive strategy (Hb ≤ 7 g/dL) for transfusion in most ICU settings. More definitive data is still required for certain specific patient populations including patients with acute neurologic injuries. Based on physiologic evidence, a higher transfusion trigger (Hb 8–9 g/dL) may be clinically acceptable in the context of critical neurologic illness, but careful individualized RBC transfusion triggers must be set according to the clinical scenario by the attending clinician until such time that rigorous evidence is available.

References

1. Bloos F, Reinhart K. Venous oximetry. Intensive Care Med. 2005;31(7):911–3.
2. Brambrink AM, Kirsch JR, editors. Essentials of neurosurgical anesthesia & critical care. New York: Springer; 2012.
3. LeRoux P. Haemoglobin management in acute brain injury. Curr Opin Crit Care. 2013;19(2):83–91.
4. Zauner A, Daugherty WP, Bullock MR, Warner DS. Brain oxygenation and energy metabolism: part I-biological function and pathophysiology. Neurosurgery. 2002;51:289–302.
5. Retter A, Wyncoll D, Pearse R, Carson D, McKechnie S, Stanworth S, et al. Guidelines on the management of anaemia and red cell transfusion in adult critically ill patients. Br J Haematol. 2013;160:445–64.
6. Hare GMT, Mazer CD, Hutchison JS, McLaren AT, Liu E, Rassouli A, et al. Severe hemodilutional anemia increases cerebral tissue injury following acute neurotrauma. J Appl Physiol. 2007;103(3):1021–9.
7. Dexter F, Hindman BJ. Effect of haemoglobin concentration on brain oxygenation in focal stroke: a mathematical modeling study. Br J Anaesth. 1997;79(3):346–51.
8. Oddo M, Milby A, Chen I, Frangos S, MacMurtrie E, Maloney-Wilensky E, et al. Hemoglobin concentration and cerebral metabolism in patients with aneurysmal subarachnoid hemorrhage. Stroke. 2009;40:1275–81.

9. Ekelund A, Reinstrup P, Ryding E, Andersson A-M, Molund T, Kristiansson K, et al. Effects of iso- and hypervolemic hemodilution on regional cerebral blood flow and oxygen delivery for patients with vasospasm after aneurysmal subarachnoid hemorrhage. Acta Neurochir (Wien). 2002;144(7):703–12; discussion 712–3.

10. Vincent JL, Baron J-F, Reinhart K, Gattinoni L, Thijs L, Webb A, et al. Anemia and blood transfusion in critically ill patients. JAMA. 2002;288(12):1499–507.

11. Walsh TS, Lee RJ, Maciver CR, Garrioch M, Mackirdy F, Binning AR, et al. Anemia during and at discharge from intensive care: the impact of restrictive blood transfusion practice. Intensive Care Med. 2006;32(1):100–9.

12. Corwin HL, Gettinger A, Pearl RG, Fink MP, Levy MM, Abraham E, et al. The CRIT Study: anemia and blood transfusion in the critically ill – current clinical practice in the United States. Crit Care Med. 2004;32(1):39–52.

13. Rosenberg NF, Koht A, Naidech AM. Anemia and transfusion after aneurysmal subarachnoid hemorrhage. J Neurosurg Anesthesiol. 2013;25(1):66–74.

14. Le Roux PD. Anemia and transfusion after subarachnoid hemorrhage. Neurocrit Care. 2011;15(2):342–53.

15. Kellert L, Schrader F, Ringleb P, Steiner T, Bösel J. The impact of low hemoglobin levels and transfusion on critical care patients with severe ischemic stroke: STroke: RelevAnt Impact of HemoGlobin, Hematocrit and Transfusion (STRAIGHT) – an observational study. J Crit Care. 2014;29(2):236–40.

16. Sampson TR, Dhar R, Diringer MN. Factors associated with the development of anemia after subarachnoid hemorrhage. Neurocrit Care. 2010;12(1):4–9.

17. Kimberly WT, Wu O, Arsava EM, Garg P, Ji R, Vangel M, et al. Lower hemoglobin correlates with larger stroke volumes in acute ischemic stroke. Cerebrovasc Dis Extra. 2011; 1(1):44–53.

18. Kellert L, Martin E, Sykora M, Bauer H, Gussmann P, Diedler J, et al. Cerebral oxygen transport failure?: decreasing hemoglobin and hematocrit levels after ischemic stroke predict poor outcome and mortality: STroke: RelevAnt Impact of hemoGlobin, Hematocrit and Transfusion (STRAIGHT) – an observational study. Stroke. 2011;42(10):2832–7.

19. Sekhon MS, McLean N, Henderson WR, Chittock DR, Griesdale DE. Association of hemoglobin concentration and mortality in critically ill patients with severe traumatic brain injury. Crit Care. 2012;16(4):R128. BioMed Central Ltd.

20. Roberts DJ, Zygun DA. Anemia, red blood cell transfusion, and outcomes after severe traumatic brain injury. Crit Care. 2012;16(5):154.

21. Oddo M, Levine JM, Kumar M, Iglesias K, Frangos S, Maloney-Wilensky E, et al. Anemia and brain oxygen after severe traumatic brain injury. Intensive Care Med. 2012;38(9):1497–504.

22. Carlson AP, Schermer CR, Lu SW. Retrospective evaluation of anemia and transfusion in traumatic brain injury. J Trauma. 2006;61(3):567–71.

23. Kuramatsu JB, Gerner ST, Lucking H, Kloska SP, Schellinger PD, Kohrmann M, et al. Anemia is an independent prognostic factor in intracerebral hemorrhage: an observational cohort study. Crit Care. 2013;17(4):R148.

24. Chang TR, Boehme AK, Aysenne A, Albright KC, Burns C, Beasley TM, et al. Nadir hemoglobin is associated with poor outcome from intracerebral hemorrhage. Springerplus. 2013;2:379.

25. Diedler J, Sykora M, Hahn P, Heerlein K, Scholzke MN, Kellert L, et al. Low hemoglobin is associated with poor functional outcome after non-traumatic, supratentorial intracerebral hemorrhage. Crit Care. 2010;14(2):R63.

26. Wartenberg KE, Mayer SA. Medical complications after subarachnoid hemorrhage: new strategies for prevention and management. Curr Opin Crit Care. 2006;12(2):78–84.

27. Kramer AH, Gurka MJ, Nathan B, Dumont AS, Kassell NF, Bleck TP. Complications associated with anemia and blood transfusion in patients with aneurysmal subarachnoid hemorrhage. Crit Care Med. 2008;36(7):2070–5.

28. Kramer AH, Zygun DA. Anemia and red blood cell transfusion in neurocritical care. Crit Care. 2009;13(3):R89.

29. Naidech AM, Drescher J, Ault ML, Shaibani A, Batjer HH, Alberts MJ. Higher hemoglobin is associated with less cerebral infarction, poor outcome, and death after subarachnoid hemorrhage. Neurosurgery. 2006;59(4):775–9; discussion 779–80.
30. Smith MJ, Stiefel MF, Magge S, Frangos S, Bloom S, Gracias V, et al. Packed red blood cell transfusion increases local cerebral oxygenation. Crit Care Med. 2005;33(5):2856; author reply 2856–7.
31. Dhar R, Scalfani M, Zazulia A, Videen T, Derdeyn C, Diringer M. Comparison of hypertension, hypervolemia, and transfusion to augment cerebral oxygen delivery after subarachnoid hemorrhage. Crit Care Med. 2010;38:A90.
32. Dhar R, Zazulia AR, Videen TO, Zipfel GJ, Derdeyn CP, Diringer MN. Red blood cell transfusion increases cerebral oxygen delivery in anemic patients with subarachnoid hemorrhage. Stroke. 2009;40(9):3039–44.
33. Dhar R, Zazulia A, Videen T, Zipfel G, Diringer M. Transfusion may be more effective at improving cerebral oxygen delivery after subarachnoid hemorrhage at lower hemoglobin levels. Neurocrit Care. 2010;13(1 Suppl):S12.
34. Hebert PC, Hu LQ, Biro GP. Review of physiologic mechanisms in response to anemia. Can Med Assoc J. 1997;156(Suppl):S27–40.
35. Creteur J, Neves AP, Vincent J-L. Near-infrared spectroscopy technique to evaluate the effects of red blood cell transfusion on tissue oxygenation. Crit Care. 2009;13 Suppl 5:S11.
36. Conrad SA, Dietrich KA, Hebert CA, Romero MD. Effect of red cell transfusion on oxygen consumption following fluid resuscitation in septic shock. Circ Shock. 1990;31(4):419–29.
37. Lorente JA, Landín L, De Pablo R, Renes E, Rodríguez-Díaz R, Liste D. Effects of blood transfusion on oxygen transport variables in severe sepsis. Crit Care Med. 1993;21(9):1312–8.
38. Marik PE, Sibbald WJ. Effect of stored-blood transfusion on oxygen delivery in patients with sepsis. JAMA. 1993;269(23):3024–9.
39. Dietrich KA, Conrad SA, Hebert CA, Levy GL, Romero MD. Cardiovascular and metabolic response to red blood cell transfusion in critically ill volume-resuscitated nonsurgical patients. Crit Care Med. 1990;18(9):940–4.
40. Casutt M, Seifert B, Pasch T, Schmid ER, Turina MI, Spahn DR. Factors influencing the individual effects of blood transfusions on oxygen delivery and oxygen consumption. Crit Care Med. 1999;27(10):2194–200.
41. Steffes CP, Bender JS, Levison MA. Blood transfusion and oxygen consumption in surgical sepsis. Crit Care Med. 1991;19(4):512–7.
42. Hébert PC, Wells G, Blajchman MA, Marshall J, Martin C, Pagliarello G, et al. A multicenter, randomized, controlled clinical trial of transfusion requirements in critical care. N Engl J Med. 1999;340(6):409–17.
43. Desjardins P, Turgeon AF, Tremblay M-H, Lauzier F, Zarychanski R, Boutin A, et al. Hemoglobin levels and transfusions in neurocritically ill patients: a systematic review of comparative studies. Crit Care. 2012;16(2):R54.
44. Jauch EC, Saver JL, Adams HP, Bruno A, Connors JJB, Demaerschalk BM, et al. Guidelines for the early management of patients with acute ischemic stroke: a guideline for healthcare professionals from the American Heart Association/American Stroke Association. Stroke. 2013;44(3):870–947.
45. Ginsberg MD, Palesch YY, Hill MD, Martin RH, Moy CS, Barsan WG, et al. High-dose albumin treatment for acute ischaemic stroke (ALIAS) part 2: a randomized, double-blind, phase 3, placebo-controlled trial. Lancet Neurol. 2013;12(11):1049–58.
46. Brain Trauma Foundation. Guidelines for the management of severe traumatic brain injury 3rd edition. J Neurotrauma. 2007;24 suppl 1:i–S106.
47. Mcintyre LA, Fergusson DA, Hutchison JS, Pagliarello G, Marshall JC. Effect of a liberal versus restrictive transfusion strategy on mortality in patients with moderate to severe head injury. Neurocrit Care. 2006;5:4–9.
48. Flückiger C, Béchir M, Brenni M, Ludwig S, Sommerfeld J, Cottini SR, et al. Increasing hematocrit above 28% during early resuscitative phase is not associated with decreased mortality following severe traumatic brain injury. Acta Neurochir (Wien). 2010;152(4):627–36.

49. George ME, Skarda DE, Watts CR, Pham HD, Beilman GJ. Aggressive red blood cell transfusion: no association with improved outcomes for victims of isolated traumatic brain injury. Neurocrit Care. 2008;8(3):337–43.
50. Warner MA, O'Keeffe T, Bhavsar P, Shringer R, Moore C, Harper C, et al. Transfusions and long-term functional outcomes in traumatic brain injury. J Neurosurg. 2010;113(3):539–46.
51. Lacroix J, Hébert PC, Hutchison JS, Hume HA, Tucci M, Ducruet T, et al. Transfusion strategies for patients in pediatric intensive care units. N Engl J Med. 2007;356(16):1609–19.
52. Morgenstern LB, Hemphill JC, Anderson C, Becker K, Broderick JP, Connolly ES, et al. Guidelines for the management of spontaneous intracerebral hemorrhage: a guideline for healthcare professionals from the American Heart Association/American Stroke Association. Stroke. 2010;41(9):2108–29.
53. Levine J, Kofke A, Cen L, Chen Z, Faerber J, Elliott JP, et al. Red blood cell transfusion is associated with infection and extracerebral complications after subarachnoid hemorrhage. Neurosurgery. 2010;66(2):312–8; discussion 318.
54. Naidech AM, Jovanovic B, Wartenberg KE, Parra A, Ostapkovich N, Connolly ES, et al. Higher hemoglobin is associated with improved outcome after subarachnoid hemorrhage. Crit Care Med. 2007;35(10):2383–9.
55. Broessner G, Lackner P, Hoefer C, Beer R, Helbok R, Grabmer C, et al. Influence of red blood cell transfusion on mortality and long-term functional outcome in 292 patients with spontaneous subarachnoid hemorrhage. Crit Care Med. 2009;37(6):1886–92.
56. Taylor C, Gough K, Gross MS J. Transfusion threshold for acute aneurysmal subarachnoid hemorrhage. J Neurosurg Anesthesiol. 2012;24(3):254–5.
57. Molyneux AJ, Kerr RSC, Yu L, Clarke M, Sneade M, Yarnold JA, et al. International subarachnoid aneurysm trial (ISAT) of neurosurgical clipping versus endovascular coiling in 2143 patients with ruptured intracranial aneurysms: a randomized comparison of effects on survival, dependency, seizures, rebleeding, subgroups, and aneurysm occlusion. Lancet. 2005; 366:809–17.
58. Connolly ES, Rabinstein AA, Carhuapoma JR, Derdeyn CP, Dion J, Higashida RT, et al. Guidelines for the management of aneurysmal subarachnoid hemorrhage: a guideline for healthcare professionals from the American Heart Association/American Stroke Association. Stroke. 2012;43(6):1711–37.
59. Tseng M-Y, Hutchinson PJ, Kirkpatrick PJ. Effects of fluid therapy following aneurysmal subarachnoid hemorrhage: a prospective clinical study. Br J Neurosurg. 2008;22(2):257–68.
60. Naidech AM, Shaibani A, Garg RK, Duran IM, Liebling SM, Bassin SL, et al. Prospective, randomized trial of higher goal hemoglobin after subarachnoid hemorrhage. Neurocrit Care. 2010;13(3):313–20.
61. Kramer AH, Diringer MN, Suarez JI, Naidech AM, Macdonald LR, Le Roux PD. Red blood cell transfusion in patients with subarachnoid hemorrhage: a multidisciplinary North American survey. Crit Care. 2011;15(1):R30.

Matthew T. Czaja and Jeffrey L. Carson

Abstract

The elderly population is growing rapidly, and the prevalence of anemia is approximately 11 % in the elderly. Observational data demonstrates poor outcome in patients with even mild anemia, but this may reflect the patients' underlying disease rather than the anemia itself. Clinical trials evaluating transfusion thresholds in the elderly suggest that a restrictive transfusion approach is safe in most clinical settings. Transfusion guidelines do not recommend specific transfusion thresholds in the elderly but rather focus on the hemoglobin level in relation to patients' comorbidities; thus, transfusion decisions may be affected by the higher prevalence of underlying medical problems in the elderly but not by age itself.

7.1 Introduction

The demographic landscape is changing at a rapid pace. Due to increases in life expectancy, the number of people aged 65 years or older is expected to rise precipitously over the next several decades. According to a 2010 report by the World Health Organization entitled "Global Health and Aging," the worldwide elderly population is projected to rise from approximately 524 million in 2010 to almost 1.5 billion by 2050. The United States is no exception to this trend; by the year 2030, an estimated 1 in 5 Americans will be elderly, representing about 72 million people. Approximately 89 million Americans will be aged 65 or older by the year 2050, more than doubling the elderly population in 2010.

Anemia is a common condition in the elderly, and thus an important consideration in the medical care of the aging population. According to the NHANES III study, the largest and most comprehensive analysis of the prevalence of anemia in the elderly, 10.6 % of community-dwelling elderly people were found to be anemic

M.T. Czaja, MD • J.L. Carson, MD (✉)
Division of General Internal Medicine, Rutgers Robert Wood Johnson Medical School, New Brunswick, NJ, USA

© Springer International Publishing Switzerland 2015
N.P. Juffermans, T.S. Walsh (eds.), *Transfusion in the Intensive Care Unit*,
DOI 10.1007/978-3-319-08735-1_7

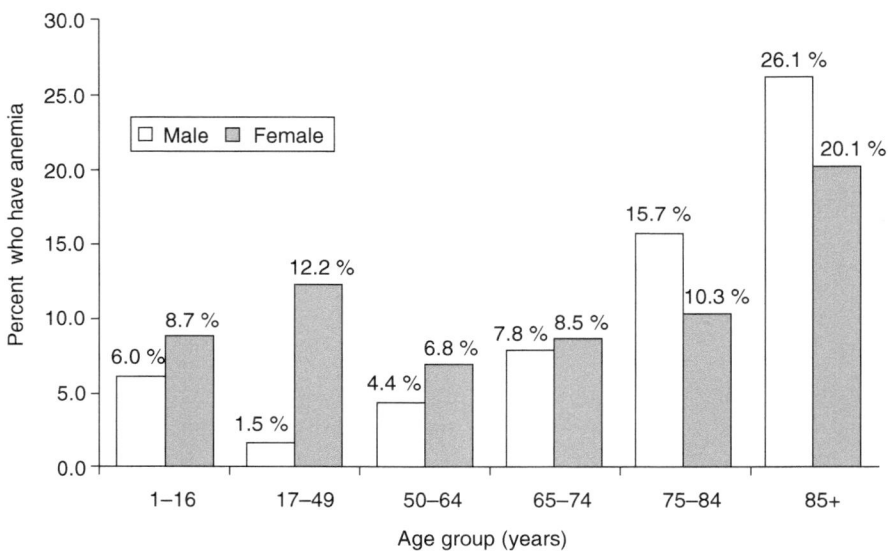

Fig. 7.1 Percentage of people with anemia according to age and sex according to NHANES III

(defined as a hemoglobin level <13 g/dL in men and <12 g/dL in women; see Fig. 7.1) [1]. The percentage of anemia in elderly men was slightly higher when compared to that of women (11.0 % vs. 10.2 %).

Furthermore, the prevalence of anemia increases steadily with age; in persons older than age 85, about one-quarter of men and one-fifth of women were anemic. These findings are similar to those of other large studies of the community-dwelling elderly population [2–4]. NHANES III also found significant differences in anemia rates in the elderly based on race and ethnicity. Non-Hispanic whites constitute the lowest prevalence (9.0 %), while non-Hispanic blacks constitute the highest (27.8 %).

Clinical data involving institutionalized elderly persons is less robust but indicates a much higher prevalence of anemia. Robinson and colleagues analyzed the charts of 6,200 nursing home residents with a mean age of 83 years old and found a 60 % prevalence of anemia [5]. Additionally, Artz et al. performed a retrospective chart review of 900 skilled nursing facility residents with a median age of 82 years old and found a mean hemoglobin of 12.9 g/dL for men and 11.9 for women [6]. The overall 6-month point prevalence of anemia was 48 %. The discrepancy in prevalence between these two studies is likely due to variations in the patient population studied, but clearly anemia is very common in the institutionalized elderly.

7.2   Etiology of Anemia in the Elderly

The causes of anemia in the elderly are generally divided into the following four categories: (1) nutrient deficiency, (2) chronic disease/inflammation, (3) chronic kidney disease, and (4) unexplained cause. NHANES III showed nearly a one-third split in prevalence between nutrient deficiencies (34 %), anemia of chronic disease (32 %), and unexplained anemia in the elderly (34 %). Half of the cases of nutrient deficiencies were due to iron deficiency (17 % of the total anemic population). Folate and vitamin B_{12} deficiency each accounted for about 6 % of all anemia. Eight percent of the cases of anemia of chronic disease were deemed secondary to chronic kidney disease. The authors theorized that the large proportion of unexplained anemia was related to the study design in that only a limited laboratory evaluation was performed in the study participants. Etiologies such as hypothyroidism, multiple myeloma, myelodysplastic syndrome, and thalassemia minor were thought to account for a significant portion of the unexplained cases.

A smaller but more intensive study performed by Price and colleagues enrolled 190 elderly patients with anemia from a hematology clinic [7]. All patients underwent a history, physical, laboratory evaluation (including a complete blood count with red cell indices, iron studies, erythropoietin level, and assessment of renal and thyroid function), and review of blood smears. Any further testing was left to the discretion of the treating physician and recorded for inclusion in the study when available. As examples, a serum protein electrophoresis was performed in 87 % of the patients, and a bone marrow biopsy was performed in 17 % of the patients. See Table 7.1 below for their results.

Table 7.1 Etiology of anemia in 190 elderly anemic patients

Etiology of anemia	Frequency (%)
Anemia of inflammation	11 (6)
Hematologic malignancy	42 (22)
Suspicious for MDS	31 (16)
MDS	7 (4)
Others	4 (2)
Iron deficiency	23 (12)
Therapy for non-hematologic malignancy	21 (11)
Renal insufficiency	8 (4)
Unexplained anemia	67 (35)
Vitamin B12 deficiency	1 (<1 %)
Folate deficiency	0 (0)
Others	11 (6)
Incomplete data	7 (4)

Despite a more thorough hematologic evaluation by Schrier et al., a similar rate of unexplained anemia was found as compared to that of NHANES III. However, the more thorough evaluation allowed for identification of several other key causes of anemia in the elderly, including hematologic malignancy and therapy for non-hematologic malignancy. A striking difference emerged between the prevalence of nutritional deficiencies between the two studies, likely due to a more stringent and accurate definition of nutritional deficiencies by Schrier et al. While the NHANES III study looked merely at blood levels of folate and vitamin B_{12} to make the diagnosis of deficiency, Schrier et al. went a step further in their definition by also requiring a hematologic response to folate or vitamin B_{12} supplementation.

7.3   Physiologic Response to Anemia in the Elderly

The human body is capable of several adaptive mechanisms in response to anemia [8]. Perhaps most importantly, the adrenergic system is ramped up in order to increase cardiac output and redirect this cardiac output to vital organs via selective arterial vasoconstriction. The renin-angiotensin-aldosterone axis is also stimulated to retain water and sodium. It is reasonable to consider that both of these hemodynamic alterations are vulnerable to attenuation with age. The incidence of heart failure increases with age, growing from about 20 per 1,000 persons between the ages of 65 and 69 to about 80 per 1,000 by age 85 or older [9]. Accordingly, the elderly may be less likely to adequately compensate to anemia by increasing cardiac output. Similar trends in rates of hypertension and peripheral vascular disease are seen with age [10], potentially making increases in vasomotor tone more difficult. This may result in reduced redirection of blood from skeletal, splanchnic, and superficial vessels to cerebral and coronary vessels that is seen in a normal compensation to anemia. All in all, elderly persons may not be able to achieve the hemodynamic changes necessary to fully compensate for anemia.

Several other age-related phenomena have been proposed as mechanisms of increased rates of anemia in the elderly. These mechanisms may also provide insight into the high rates of unexplained anemia seen in the studies mentioned above. Makipour et al. theorized that the following factors may contribute to anemia in the elderly [11]:

1. Age-related decline in renal function, resulting in decreased erythropoietin levels.
2. Age-related decline in androgen levels, which has been shown to correlate with a decrease in hemoglobin. For instance, the InCHIANTI study found an association between low testosterone and anemia in an elderly Italian population without cancer or chronic kidney disease [12].
3. Increased prevalence of chronic inflammatory conditions in the elderly, such as cancer, arthritis, atherosclerosis, and others.
4. Though still under investigation, there is growing evidence that hematopoietic stem cells lose proliferative and regenerative function over time [13, 14].

It is worthy to note that another major compensation for anemia is a shift to the right in the oxyhemoglobin dissociation curve. This is made possible by increased production of 2,3-diphosphoglycerate in red blood cells, which results in increased oxygen delivery to tissues at a given partial pressure of oxygen. After a literature search, no recent studies were found that specifically address the effect of aging on the oxyhemoglobin dissociation curve.

7.4   Consequences of Anemia in the Elderly

A review of the literature of the adverse consequences of anemia in the elderly can be broadly divided by the outcomes that were studied. Functional ability, cognitive function, and mortality are three of the most common outcomes studied in this population and are reviewed below. It is important to note that in studies that found worse outcomes in anemic elderly patients, it remains unknown if the anemia itself or the underlying cause of the anemia and/or associated comorbidities is the culprit. We suspect that the underlying cause and comorbidity are responsible for worse outcomes rather than anemia itself.

A number of studies found an association between anemia in the elderly and poor functional status [15–18]. Penninx et al. studied a cohort of 1,146 anemic elderly patients by assessing various markers of physical performance, including a standing balance test, a timed 8-foot walk, and a timed test of 5 chair rises [17]. After adjustment for patients' baseline performance scores, age, sex, cigarette smoking, blood pressure, and comorbid conditions, anemia was associated with a statistically significant decline in physical performance when compared to a control group. Additionally, separate studies by Penninx et al. showed decreased handgrip and knee extension strength [18] and a higher risk of falls [19] in the anemic elderly.

In addition to its effect on physical performance, anemia in the elderly has been shown to impact cognitive function as well. The Women's Health and Aging Study showed an association between mild anemia (hemoglobin 10–12 g/dL) and lower executive function in high-functioning, community-dwelling elderly women [20]. In the "Health and Anemia" study, researchers found that anemic elderly persons performed worse on a host of cognitive testing but, after adjustment for possible cofounders, only selective attention remained statistically significant [21]. Hong and colleagues utilized the Health, Aging, and Body Composition study, a prospective cohort of community-dwelling persons aged 70–79, to study the association between anemia and the risk of dementia [22]. Out of 2,552 study participants with available hemoglobin levels, 393 (15 %) were diagnosed with anemia. After 11 years of follow-up, dementia was diagnosed in 23 % of the anemic patients versus 17 % on non-anemic controls. These results remained statistically significant after adjustment for several variables including comorbid conditions. Two earlier studies found similar results with smaller groups of patients and a shorter follow-up period [23, 24].

The most important question is whether anemia in the elderly affects mortality rates. In a study of 755 persons aged 85 and above, risk of mortality was 1.60 (95 %

confidence interval, 1.24–2.06; $P<.001$) in women with anemia and 2.29 (95 % confidence interval, 1.60–3.26; $P<.001$) in men with anemia after 5 years of follow-up, a finding that remained similar after adjustment for known diseases at baseline [25]. Higher mortality due to malignant neoplasms and infections was found in the anemic cohort. Of note, there was no difference in mortality found from years 5 to 10 of the study.

Mortality in relation to anemia in the elderly was also analyzed using the Cardiovascular Health Study, a cohort of 5,888 community-dwelling elderly persons [4]. After about 11 years of follow-up, mortality rates for those with and without anemia were 57 and 39 %, respectively ($P<0.001$). Similarly, the Populations for Epidemiologic Studies of the Elderly cohort was used to show a relative risk of death of 1.61 (95 % confidence interval, 1.34–1.93) when comparing 451 elderly anemic persons to non-anemic persons after adjustment for demographics and baseline comorbidities. This finding remained statistically significant after excluding all patients with certain chronic medical conditions at the onset of the study [26].

7.5 Randomized Controlled Trials of Blood Transfusion in the Elderly

Few large, randomized controlled trials exist on blood transfusions in the elderly. The FOCUS trial by Carson et al., a study of blood transfusions in the postoperative period, provides insight into this question in that nearly all the patients in the study were elderly [27]. This multicenter randomized clinical trial enrolled 2,016 patients aged 50 years or older who underwent surgical repair of a hip fracture with a postoperative hemoglobin level of less than 10 g/dL. Only patients with cardiovascular disease (i.e., history of ischemic heart disease, congestive heart failure, transient ischemic attack, stroke, or peripheral vascular disease or electrocardiographic evidence of a previous myocardial infarction) or cardiovascular risk factors (i.e., hypertension, diabetes mellitus, tobacco history, or a creatinine level above 2.0 mg/dL) were included in the study.

Participants were randomized to either the liberal-strategy or the restrictive-strategy group. In the liberal-strategy group, patients were transfused with blood until their hemoglobin level reached 10 g/dL. Patients in the restrictive-strategy group received blood transfusions at the discretion of the treating physicians to maintain a hemoglobin level above 8 g/dL or for symptoms consistent with anemia (e.g., cardiac chest pain, hypotension, tachycardia, and congestive heart failure). Transfusion was permitted at any time regardless of the hemoglobin level if blood transfusion was deemed necessary to treat active bleeding.

The primary outcome of the FOCUS trial was mortality or an inability to walk 10 ft without human assistance at 60 days. Secondary outcomes included a composite of in-hospital myocardial infarction, unstable angina, or death from any reason. Baseline characteristics were similar between the two groups. The mean age of the study population was 81.6 years. Cardiovascular disease was present in 63 % of the participants, including 40 % with coronary artery disease and about 17 % with congestive heart failure. The median number of units of blood transfused was 2.0 in the liberal-strategy group and 0 in the restrictive-strategy group. The liberal-strategy group had a 1.3 g/dL higher hemoglobin level prior to transfusion as compared to that of the restrictive-strategy group. Almost 60 % of the patients in the restrictive-strategy group did not receive a blood transfusion.

The results showed an odds ratio of 1.01 (95 % confidence interval, 0.84–1.22) comparing the primary outcome (death or inability to walk 10 ft without human assistance at 60 days) in the liberal-strategy group (35.2 %) versus the restrictive-strategy group (34.7 %). Interactions according to age were not significant. Furthermore, the difference in mortality at 30 days was not statistically significant (5.2 % in the liberal-strategy group and 4.3 % in the restrictive-strategy group) nor were the rates of in-hospital myocardial infarction or unstable angina.

Overall, no evidence was found to support maintaining a postoperative hemoglobin level above 10 g/dL as compared to 8 g/dL. The authors note that a "high-risk group of patients with a mean age of more than 81 years" was enrolled, a population "for whom untreated anemia would probably be more harmful than in a healthier or younger population undergoing most surgical procedures." In other words, despite the old age and high prevalence of cardiovascular disease and other comorbidities, no change in functional ability, mortality, or morbidity was found in a population who may be expected to benefit most from increased hemoglobin- and oxygen-carrying capacity.

The TRICC study performed by Hébert et al. [28] also adds to our knowledge of blood transfusion in the elderly. This randomized, controlled, clinical trial examined a restrictive versus liberal transfusion strategy in 838 critically ill patients across 25 hospitals in Canada in the mid-1990s. Patients were included if they were expected to stay in the intensive care unit for more than 24 h, had a hemoglobin level of 9 g/dL or less within 3 days of admission to the intensive care unit, and were considered euvolemic by their treating physicians. Key exclusion criteria included major active blood loss (a decrease in hemoglobin of 3.0 g/dL or more in the preceding 12 h) and chronic anemia with a hemoglobin level less than 9.0 g/dL.

Patients were then randomized to the liberal- or restrictive-strategy group after being stratified by their APACHE II score. In the liberal-strategy group, patients were transfused to maintain a hemoglobin of at least 10 g/dL with a goal hemoglobin of 10–12 g/dL. Conversely, the goal hemoglobin in the restrictive-strategy group was 7–9 g/dL, such that transfusion was indicated for a hemoglobin less than 7.0 g/dL. Suggestions for the use of intravenous fluids and vasoactive medications were provided but all management decisions were left to the discretion of the treating physicians.

The primary outcome was death from all causes in the first 30 days after randomization, and secondary outcomes included 60-day rates of death from all causes, death during the intensive care unit stay and during hospitalization, and survival times in the first 30 days. The two groups were similar in terms of baseline characteristics. The average age was 57–58 years old. Adherence to the study protocol was excellent. The average daily hemoglobin concentration was 8.5 g/dL in the restrictive-strategy group as compared to 10.7 g/dL in the liberal-strategy group ($P < 0.01$). Accordingly, patients in the restrictive-strategy group received an average of 3 fewer red cell units.

Fig. 7.2 Kaplan-Meier estimate of survival in the 30 days after admission to the intensive care unit in the restrictive versus liberal-strategy groups (adapted)

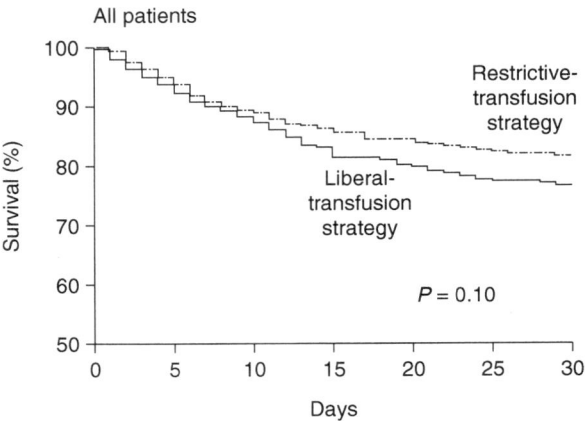

At the end of the study, the primary outcome (rate of death from all causes after 30 days) was 18.7 % in the restrictive-strategy group and 23.3 % in the liberal-strategy group ($P=0.11$; Fig. 7.2). The authors also analyzed a prespecified subgroup of patients 55 years or older as these patients were thought to potentially suffer worse outcomes due to a decreased ability to compensate for anemia. The subgroup of patients >55 years old did not differ significantly in their baseline characteristics from those of younger patients. All outcomes between the two transfusion strategies in older patients were similar. Of note, in patients under the age of 55, the 30-day mortality rate was significantly higher in the liberal-strategy group (13.0 % vs. 5.7 %, $P=0.02$).

All in all, while TRICC used a cutoff age of 55 years old, the study failed to show that older adults benefit from a higher hemoglobin level derived from a liberal transfusion strategy.

7.6   Clinical Guidelines on Blood Transfusion in the Elderly

The majority of professional society guidelines on blood transfusions do not incorporate age into their recommendations. For example, the AABB (formerly the American Association of Blood Banks) guidelines, perhaps the most widely used set of recommendations, do not explicitly mention the elderly in their recommendations [29]. However, the authors note that "clinical trials are needed in other patient populations that include…elderly medical patients recovering from illnesses that result in hospitalization…." The "Clinical practice guideline: Red blood cell transfusion in adult trauma and critical care," published in *Critical Care Medicine* in 2009, also does not explicitly mention age as a consideration [30]. Other examples of guidelines that fail to specifically comment on the elderly include the 2013 clinical practice guideline of treatment of anemia in patients with heart disease by the American College of Physicians [31] and "Guidelines for transfusion in the trauma patient" by West et al. published in the *Journal of Trauma* [32].

When mentioned, age is generally considered a small piece of the puzzle in the decision-making process of transfusing blood. Guidelines published in 2001 in the *British Journal of Haematology* briefly allude to anemia in the elderly in the following statement: "In patients who may tolerate anaemia poorly, e.g. patients over the age of 65 years,…consider adopting a higher concentration at which transfusions are indicated, e.g. when the haemoglobin concentration becomes <8 g/dL" [33].

Similarly, the International Society of Nephrology guidelines on anemia in patients with chronic kidney disease (CKD) reference anemia in the elderly very briefly [34]. In the section entitled "Use of erythropoiesis-stimulating agents and other agents to treat anemia in CKD," the authors generally recommend a hemoglobin goal of 10 g/dL in the adult patient with CKD. However, the authors go on to caution readers that in certain subsets of patients with CKD stages III–V, it "may not be wise" to allow the hemoglobin level to drift below 10 g/dL, especially in "elderly patients who are more prone to developing symptoms and signs of anemia."

The Society of Thoracic Surgeons and the Society of Cardiovascular Anesthesiologists Clinical Practice Guidelines, published in the *Annals of Thoracic Surgeons* in 2012, discuss anemia in the elderly [35]. Ferraris et al. note that several factors contribute to an increased risk of bleeding and the subsequent need for blood transfusion (such as advanced age, preoperative anemia, small body size, multiple comorbidities, etc.). The authors reason that such patients should be identified prior to surgery and "all available preoperative and perioperative measures of blood conservation should be undertaken in this group." They go on to assert that while these high-risk patient factors are listed as single factors that are either present or absent, many of them represent a spectrum of severity. Age is used as an example of this assertion in that "the risk [of bleeding and the need for blood transfusion] associated with age greater than 75 years is significantly greater than the risk for a patient aged 55 years or younger, and it is quite likely that the risk of transfusion associated with age is not a continuous function."

7.7 Conclusion

Given the rapid pace of aging in the population and the increased prevalence of anemia with age, anemia in the elderly is an important topic of consideration. The etiology of anemia in this population remains puzzling as high rates of unexplained anemia have been found. Furthermore, it is theorized that the elderly are less able to tolerate anemia due to their inability to mount an adequate physiologic response as compared to that of younger persons. Observational data has shown that anemia is associated with worse outcomes in the elderly, including an increase in mortality. However, given the increased prevalence of diseases such as coronary artery disease, congestive heart failure, chronic kidney disease, and cancer in the elderly, such studies are unable to determine if anemia is the true cause of adverse outcomes or merely a marker of underlying comorbidity. Randomized controlled trials such as the TRICC and FOCUS studies, which included a large proportion of elderly patients with cardiovascular disease and risk factors, did not show evidence that a liberal versus restrictive blood transfusion strategy improves outcomes. Major society guidelines have not set forth specific recommendations on the topic of adopting a restrictive versus liberal blood transfusion strategy in the elderly, a result of the lack of randomized clinical trials that specifically address the subject.

All in all, anemia is a common disease affecting the elderly and has been shown in observational data to portend worse outcomes, but there is no evidence to incorporate age itself in developing a blood transfusion strategy.

References

1. Guralnik JM, Eisenstaedt RS, Ferrucci L, Klein HG, Woodman RC. Prevalence of anemia in persons 65 years and older in the United States: evidence for a high rate of unexplained anemia. Blood. 2004;104:2263–8.
2. Inelmen EM, D'Alessio M, Gatto MR, et al. Descriptive analysis of the prevalence of anemia in a randomly selected sample of elderly people living at home: some results of an Italian multicentric study. Aging (Milan, Italy). 1994;6:81–9.
3. Salive ME, Cornoni-Huntley J, Guralnik JM, et al. Anemia and hemoglobin levels in older persons: relationship with age, gender, and health status. J Am Geriatr Soc. 1992;40:489–96.
4. Zakai NA, Katz R, Hirsch C, et al. A prospective study of anemia status, hemoglobin concentration, and mortality in an elderly cohort: the cardiovascular health study. Arch Intern Med. 2005;165:2214–20.
5. Robinson B, Artz AS, Culleton B, Critchlow C, Sciarra A, Audhya P. Prevalence of anemia in the nursing home: contribution of chronic kidney disease. J Am Geriatr Soc. 2007;55:1566–70.
6. Artz AS, Fergusson D, Drinka PJ, et al. Prevalence of anemia in skilled-nursing home residents. Arch Gerontol Geriatr. 2004;39:201–6.
7. Price EA, Mehra R, Holmes TH, Schrier SL. Anemia in older persons: etiology and evaluation. Blood Cells Mol Dis. 2011;46:159–65.
8. Hebert PC, Van der Linden P, Biro G, Hu LQ. Physiologic aspects of anemia. Crit Care Clin. 2004;20:187–212.
9. Curtis LH, Whellan DJ, Hammill BG, et al. Incidence and prevalence of heart failure in elderly persons, 1994-2003. Arch Intern Med. 2008;168:418–24.
10. Members WG, Roger VL, Go AS, et al. Heart disease and stroke statistics—2012 update: a report from the American Heart Association. Circulation. 2012;125:e2–220.
11. Makipour S, Kanapuru B, Ershler WB. Unexplained anemia in the elderly. Semin Hematol. 2008;45:250–4.
12. Ferrucci L, Maggio M, Bandinelli S, et al. Low testosterone levels and the risk of anemia in older men and women. Arch Intern Med. 2006;166:1380–8.
13. Rossi DJ, Jamieson CHM, Weissman IL. Stems cells and the pathways to aging and cancer. Cell. 2008;132:681–96.
14. Dumble M, Moore L, Chambers SM, et al. The impact of altered p53 dosage on hematopoietic stem cell dynamics during aging. Blood. 2007;109:1736–42.
15. Chaves PH, Semba RD, Leng SX, et al. Impact of anemia and cardiovascular disease on frailty status of community-dwelling older women: the Women's Health and Aging Studies I and II. J Gerontol A Biol Sci Med Sci. 2005;60:729–35.
16. Chaves PH, Ashar B, Guralnik JM, Fried LP. Looking at the relationship between hemoglobin concentration and prevalent mobility difficulty in older women. Should the criteria currently used to define anemia in older people be reevaluated? J Am Geriatr Soc. 2002;50:1257–64.
17. Penninx BW, Guralnik JM, Onder G, Ferrucci L, Wallace RB, Pahor M. Anemia and decline in physical performance among older persons. Am J Med. 2003;115:104–10.

18. Penninx BW, Pahor M, Cesari M, et al. Anemia is associated with disability and decreased physical performance and muscle strength in the elderly. J Am Geriatr Soc. 2004;52:719–24.
19. Penninx BW, Pluijm SM, Lips P, et al. Late-life anemia is associated with increased risk of recurrent falls. J Am Geriatr Soc. 2005;53:2106–11.
20. Chaves PH, Carlson MC, Ferrucci L, Guralnik JM, Semba R, Fried LP. Association between mild anemia and executive function impairment in community-dwelling older women: The Women's Health and Aging Study II. J Am Geriatr Soc. 2006;54:1429–35.
21. Lucca U, Tettamanti M, Mosconi P, et al. Association of mild anemia with cognitive, functional mood and quality of life outcomes in the elderly: the "Health and Anemia" study. PLoS One. 2008;3:e1920.
22. Hong CH, Falvey C, Harris TB, et al. Anemia and risk of dementia in older adults: findings from the Health ABC study. Neurology. 2013;81:528–33.
23. Atti AR, Palmer K, Volpato S, Zuliani G, Winblad B, Fratiglioni L. Anaemia increases the risk of dementia in cognitively intact elderly. Neurobiol Aging. 2006;27:278–84.
24. Shah RC, Buchman AS, Wilson RS, Leurgans SE, Bennett DA. Hemoglobin level in older persons and incident Alzheimer disease: prospective cohort analysis. Neurology. 2011;77:219–26.
25. Izaks GJ, Westendorp RG, Knook DL. The definition of anemia in older persons. JAMA. 1999;281:1714–7.
26. Penninx BW, Pahor M, Woodman RC, Guralnik JM. Anemia in old age is associated with increased mortality and hospitalization. J Gerontol A Biol Sci Med Sci. 2006;61:474–9.
27. Carson JL, Terrin ML, Noveck H, et al. Liberal or restrictive transfusion in high-risk patients after hip surgery. N Engl J Med. 2011;365:2453–62.
28. Hébert PC, Wells G, Blajchman MA, et al. A multicenter, randomized, controlled clinical trial of transfusion requirements in critical care. N Engl J Med. 1999;340:409–17.
29. Carson JL, Grossman BJ, Kleinman S, et al. Red blood cell transfusion: a clinical practice guideline from the AABB*. Ann Intern Med. 2012;157:49–58.
30. Napolitano LM, Kurek S, Luchette FA, et al. Clinical practice guideline: red blood cell transfusion in adult trauma and critical care. J Trauma. 2009;67:1439–42.
31. Qaseem A, Humphrey LL, Fitterman N, Starkey M, Shekelle P. Treatment of anemia in patients with heart disease: a clinical practice guideline from the American College of Physicians. Ann Intern Med. 2013;159:770–9.
32. West MA, Shapiro MB, Nathens AB, et al. Inflammation and the host response to injury, a large-scale collaborative project: patient-oriented research core–standard operating procedures for clinical care: IV. Guidelines for transfusion in the trauma patient. J Trauma Acute Care Surg. 2006;61:436–9. doi:10.1097/01.ta.0000232517.83039.c4.
33. Murphy MF, Wallington TB, Kelsey P, Boulton F, Bruce M, Cohen H, Duguid J, Knowles SM, Poole G, Williamson LM, British Committee for Standards in Haematology, Blood Transfusion Task Force. Guidelines for the clinical use of red cell transfusions. Br J Haematol. 2001;113:24–31.
34. Kidney Disease: Improving Global Outcomes (KDIGO) Anemia Work Group. KDIGO clinical practice guideline for anemia in chronic kidney disease. Kidney Int Suppl. 2012;2:279–335.
35. Ferraris VA, Ferraris SP, Saha SP, et al. Perioperative blood transfusion and blood conservation in cardiac surgery: the Society of Thoracic Surgeons and The Society of Cardiovascular Anesthesiologists clinical practice guideline. Ann Thorac Surg. 2007;83:S27–86.

ScvO₂ as an Alternative Transfusion Trigger

Szilvia Kocsi, Krisztián Tánczos, and Zsolt Molnár

Abstract

Blood transfusion is often a life-saving but risky intervention. Restrictive transfusion protocols have recently been developed with a post-transfusion target haemoglobin level of 7–10 g/dL. Whether only haemoglobin level is enough to guide our transfusion practice is questionable; hence, the same level of anaemia may be harmless in sedated, haemodynamically stable patients, while it requires urgent treatment in unstable patients or when oxygen demand is increased. Therefore, it is not the haemoglobin level *per se* that determines the severity of anaemia but the imbalance between oxygen delivery and consumption. One of the simple surrogates to estimate the balance of the oxygen extraction ratio is central venous oxygen saturation. In this chapter, the role of central venous oxygen saturation as an alternative transfusion trigger in addition to haemoglobin will be discussed.

8.1 Introduction

Oxygen is essential for sustaining life; therefore, it is of crucial importance in the critically ill to deliver adequate oxygen to the tissues to meet their metabolic requirements. When impairment arises between oxygen delivery and consumption due to anaemia, blood transfusion may be needed. Untreated anaemia can be associated with increased morbidity and mortality, while transfusion may

S. Kocsi
Department of Anaesthesiology and Intensive Therapy, Hungarian Defence Forces Military Hospital, Robert Karoly Korut 44, Budapest 1134, Hungary

K. Tánczos • Z. Molnár (✉)
Department of Anaesthesiology and Intensive Therapy, University of Szeged, Semmelweis Utca 6, Szeged 6725, Hungary
e-mail: zsoltmolna@gmail.com

© Springer International Publishing Switzerland 2015
N.P. Juffermans, T.S. Walsh (eds.), *Transfusion in the Intensive Care Unit*,
DOI 10.1007/978-3-319-08735-1_8

cause various infectious and non-infectious adverse effects [1–4]. A number of guidelines have been published to help transfusion practice; however, the criteria for the optimal management of anaemia are not clearly defined. In most guidelines, the indication of blood transfusion is based on a certain level of haemoglobin, usually 7–10 g/dL [2, 5, 6].

One of the landmark studies in the field, the TRICC (Transfusion Requirement in Critical Care) trial, found no benefit with the use of a liberal transfusion strategy to maintain haemoglobin (Hb) levels of 10 g/dL as compared with a restrictive approach where transfusions were only indicated to patients with a haemoglobin level <7 g/dL [2]. However, this should not be applied as a generalised concept, because it may hold true for a population, but cannot be applied for every individual patient. Therefore, in order to determine individualised transfusion triggers, we need to consider physiological indicators of blood transfusion based on anaemia-caused oxygen debt.

8.2   Anaemia and Oxygen Debt

The adequacy of tissue oxygenation is determined by the balance between the rate of oxygen transport to the tissues (oxygen delivery, DO_2) and the rate at which the oxygen is used by the tissues (oxygen consumption, VO_2) [7]. Standard formulae to determine oxygen delivery and oxygen consumption are

$$DO_2 = SV \times HR \times \left[Hb \times 1.34 \times SaO_2 + 0.003 \times PaO_2 \right] = CO \times \left[CaO_2 \right]$$

$$VO_2 = SV \times HR \times \left[CaO_2 - \left(Hb \times 1.34 \times SvO_2 + 0.003 \times PvO_2 \right) \right] = CO \times \left[CaO_2 - CvO_2 \right]$$

DO_2, oxygen delivery; SV, stroke volume; HR, heart rate; Hb, haemoglobin; SaO_2, arterial haemoglobin oxygen saturation; PaO_2, arterial oxygen partial pressure; CO, cardiac output; CaO_2, arterial oxygen content; VO_2, oxygen consumption; SvO_2, mixed venous haemoglobin oxygen saturation; PvO_2, mixed venous oxygen partial pressure; CvO_2, mixed venous oxygen content

From the above formulae, oxygen delivery for an average adult at rest can be calculated:

$$CO = 70 \, mL \times 72 \, / \, min = 5 \, L \, / \, min$$

$$CaO_2 = \left(150 \, g \, / \, L \times 1.34 \, mL \times 1 \right) + \left(0.003 \times 100 \, mmHg \right) = 201.3 \, mL \, / \, L$$

$$DO_2 \sim 1000 \, mL \, / \, min$$

Oxygen consumption at rest is

$$CvO_2 = \left(150 \, g \, / \, L \times 1.34 \, mL \times 0.75 \right) + \left(0.003 \times 40 \, mmHg \right) = 150.87$$

$$VO_2 = 5 \, L \, / \, min \times \left(201.3 \, mL \, / \, L - 150.87 \, mL \, / \, L \right) \sim 250 \, mL \, / \, min$$

$$\text{Oxygen extraction} \left(VO_2 / DO_2 \times 100 \right) = 250 \, mL / min / 1000 \, mL / min \times 100 = 25\%$$

In the critically ill, there is often an imbalance between delivery and consumption: DO_2 may be too low for several reasons (hypovolaemia, bleeding, pump failure, etc.) and frequently accompanied by increased VO_2 (agitation, fever, pain, etc.). The circulation can compensate to some extent, but after a critical threshold severe oxygen debt and shock may occur [8].

One of the most common causes of inadequate DO_2 in the intensive care unit is anaemia requiring red blood cell transfusions [9]. It has recently been suggested that haemoglobin level should not be the only factor on which the indication of transfusion is based [5, 6]. Clinicians utilise different tools from simple clinical signs (confusion, tachycardia, ST segment elevation/depression, diuresis) to invasive haemodynamic measurements (central venous oxygen saturation, oxygen extraction, central venous-to-arterial carbon dioxide difference) in order to have information on anaemia-related altered oxygen extraction and hence the need for blood administration [10]. One of the potentially useful physiological parameters is the central venous oxygen saturation ($ScvO_2$).

8.3   Central Venous Oxygen Saturation (ScvO$_2$) as a Transfusion Trigger

$ScvO_2$ is an easily obtained parameter via the central venous catheter already *in situ* in most critically ill patients, and it is often used as a marker of the balance between oxygen delivery and consumption. The normal value of $ScvO_2$ varies between 73 and 82 % [6, 7]. It is slightly higher than mixed venous oxygen saturation (SvO_2) and is considered a reasonable surrogate marker in the clinical setting [10]. The main factors which influence $ScvO_2$ are haemoglobin, arterial oxygen saturation of haemoglobin, cardiac output and oxygen consumption (Fig. 8.1).

It was found during haemorrhage in animal and human experimental models that $ScvO_2$ may be useful for the identification of patients with occult or ongoing clinically significant blood loss [11, 12]. In bleeding conditions, a $ScvO_2$ value of ~70 % has been used as a goal to therapeutic intervention in attempts at improving oxygen delivery [10]. In a prospective human interventional study, it was found that acute isovolaemic anaemia with a haemoglobin of 5 g/dL in conscious healthy resting humans did not produce haemodynamic instability, but oxygen imbalance was accompanied by a significant drop in mixed venous saturation [13]. These results were reinforced by a retrospective analysis of a prospective observational study in which $ScvO_2$ was found to be a good indicator of transfusion [14]. The results of our recent animal study on isovolaemic haemodilution gave further evidence that anaemia-induced change in oxygen balance can be monitored by $ScvO_2$ [15]. We found a strong, negative correlation between VO_2/DO_2 and $ScvO_2$ ($r = -0.71$, $p < 0.001$). Taking >30 % as the

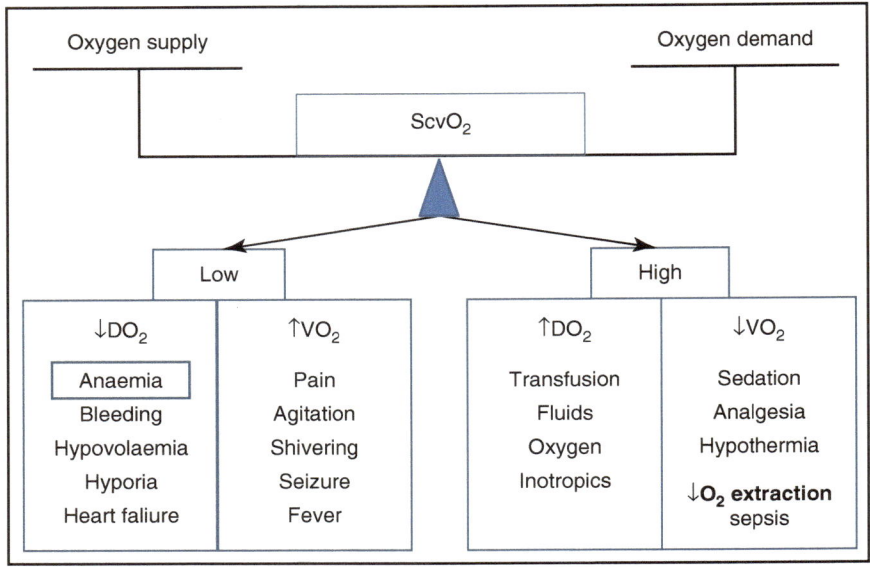

Fig. 8.1 Factors affecting $ScvO_2$

critical threshold of VO_2/DO_2 for indicating oxygen debt, the area under the curve (AUC) for $ScvO_2$ was compelling (AUC = 0.768 ± 0.056 ($0.657–0.878$) $p < 0.001$).

These results suggest that $ScvO_2$ may help to identify the point when compensatory mechanisms become exhausted and the relationship between VO_2 and DO_2 tips the balance; hence, transfusion is indicated as compared to the haemoglobin concentration alone. In clinical practice, "low" haemoglobin levels do not necessarily lead to oxygen debt in haemodynamically stable, anaesthetised, ventilated patients, while oxygen imbalance may occur in agitated, pyrexial patients with "higher" haemoglobin levels. These findings are also in accord with the physiology that compensatory changes in cardiac output and other parameters of oxygen delivery make haemoglobin concentration alone a less sensitive marker of oxygen balance and for the need for therapeutic intervention to increase DO_2.

Therefore, we believe that in addition to the haemoglobin levels, whenever feasible, $ScvO_2$ in the context of other clinical signs of altered oxygen demand (confusion, angina, low diuresis, serum lactate level, etc.) should be taken into account before administering red blood cells to patients, in order to reduce the number of unnecessary transfusions and transfusion-related complications.

8.4   Conclusion

Blood transfusion in general has been and will most probably remain a life-saving intervention for decades to come. Thorough understanding of the details of physiology, especially the relationship between oxygen delivery and consumption, is of utmost importance, even in transfusion practice. With the help of an easily obtainable physiological indicator, such as the ScvO$_2$, we can individualise our transfusion protocols, thence apply safe care for our patients.

References

1. Vincent JL, Piagnerelli M. Transfusion in the intensive care unit. Crit Care Med. 2006;34:96–101.
2. Hébert PC, Wells G, Blajchman MA, Marshall J, Martin C, Pagliarello G, Tweddale M, Schweitzer I, Yetisir E. A multicenter, randomized, controlled clinical trial of transfusion requirements in critical care. N Engl J Med. 1999;340:409–17.
3. Galvin I, Ferguson ND. Acute lung injury in the ICU: focus on prevention. In: Vincent JL, editor. Annual update in intensive care and emergency medicine 2011. New York: Springer; 2011. p. 117–28.
4. Vlaar AP, Juffermans NP. Transfusion-related acute lung injury: a clinical review. Lancet. 2013;382:984–94.
5. Westbrook A, Pettilä V, Nichol A, Bailey MJ, Syres G, Murray L, Bellomo R, Wood E, Phillips LE, Street A, French C, Orford N, Santamaria J, Cooper DJ. Transfusion practice and guidelines in Australian and New Zealand intensive care units. Intensive Care Med. 2010;36:1138–46.
6. Vallet B, Robin E, Lebuffe G. Venous oxygen saturation as a physiologic transfusion trigger. Crit Care. 2010;14:213.
7. Vallet B, Tavernier B, Lund N. Assessment of tissue oxygenation in the critically ill. Eur J Anaesthesiol. 2000;17:221–9.
8. Reinhardt K, Bloos F. The value of venous oximetry. Curr Opin Crit Care. 2005;11:259–63.
9. Gattinoni L, Chiumello D. Anemia in the intensive care unit: how big is the problem? Transfus Altern Transfus Med. 2002;4:118–20.
10. Bracht H, Eigenmann V, Haenggi M, Inderbitzin D, Jakob SM, Loher S, et al. Perioperative ScvO$_2$ monitoring. Multicentre study on peri- and postoperative central venous oxygen saturation in high-risk surgical patients. Crit Care. 2006;10:158.
11. Scalea TM, Holman M, Fuortes M, Baron BJ, Phillips TF, Goldstein AS, Sclafani SJ, Shaftan GW. Central venous–blood oxygen saturation–an early, accurate measurement of volume during hemorrhage. J Trauma 1988;28:725–32.
12. Pearse R, Dawson D, Fawcett J, Rhodes A, Grounds RM, Bennett ED. Changes in central venous saturation after major surgery, and association with outcome. Crit Care. 2005;9:694–9.
13. Weisskopff RB, Viele MK, Feiner JB, et al. Human cardiovascular and metabolic response to severe, isovolaemic anaemia. JAMA 1988;279:217–21.
14. Adamczyk S, Robin E, Barreau O, Fleyfel M, Tavernier B, Lebuffe G, Vallet B. Contribution of central venous oxygen saturation in postoperative blood transfusion decision. Ann Fr Anesth Reanim 2009;28:522–30.
15. Kocsi S, Demeter G, Fogas J, Érces D, Kaszaki J, Molnár Z. Central venous oxygen saturation is a good indicator of altered oxygen balance in isovolemic anemia. Acta Anaesthesiol Scand. 2012;56:291–7.

Howard L. Corwin and Lena M. Napolitano

Abstract

Anemia is common in the critically ill and patients with anemia tend to have worse clinical outcomes. Red blood cell transfusion as a treatment for anemia is associated with risk but little evidence of clinical benefit. As a consequence, alternatives to red blood cell transfusion for the treatment of anemia in the critically ill have been sought. This chapter will examine the clinical evidence regarding the current status of iron supplementation, erythropoietin-stimulating agents, and hemoglobin-based oxygen carriers in the treatment of anemia in the critically ill.

9.1 Introduction

Anemia is common in the critically ill with almost 95 % of patients demonstrating some level of anemia by ICU day 3 [1]. This anemia persists following ICU discharge with a median time to recovery of 11 weeks, and 53 % of patients still anemic 6 months after ICU discharge [2]. The etiology of anemia in the critically ill, while multifactorial, has been referred to as anemia of inflammation (AI), reflecting the crucial role of the inflammatory process in the pathophysiology of the anemia in this clinical setting [3].

For much of the last century, red blood cell (RBC) transfusions were viewed as a safe and effective means of treating anemia and improving oxygen delivery to tissues. Beginning in the early 1980s, primarily driven by the risk of transfusion-related infection, RBC transfusion practice began to come under scrutiny. What

H.L. Corwin, MD (✉)
Department of Medicine, University of Arkansas for Medical Sciences,
Little Rock, AR 72205, USA
e-mail: hcorwin@uams.edu

L.M. Napolitano, MD
Department of Surgery, University of Michigan Health System, Ann Arbor, MI, USA

© Springer International Publishing Switzerland 2015   77
N.P. Juffermans, T.S. Walsh (eds.), *Transfusion in the Intensive Care Unit*,
DOI 10.1007/978-3-319-08735-1_9

started as primarily a concern over the risks of RBC transfusion, over the last two decades, has shifted to include a more critical examination of the benefits of RBC transfusion. Numerous studies over the past two decades have failed to demonstrate a benefit to RBC transfusion in many of the clinical situations in which RBC transfusions are routinely given and in fact have shown that RBC transfusion can lead to worse clinical outcomes in some patients [4, 5]. The few available large, randomized, clinical trials and prospective observational studies that have assessed the effectiveness of allogeneic RBC transfusion have demonstrated that a more restrictive approach to RBC transfusion results to at least equivalent patient outcomes compared to a liberal approach and may actually reduce morbidity and mortality rates [4, 5]. To date, there are no convincing data to support the routine use of RBC transfusion to treat anemia in hemodynamically stable critically ill patients without evidence of acute bleeding. Over the last decade, RBC transfusion best-practice guidelines have been developed by a number of professional societies [6] addressing RBC transfusion practice in specific patient populations including critical care. These guidelines are generally consistent, strongly recommending a restrictive RBC transfusion approach in most clinical populations.

The observations that anemia in critically ill patients is associated with poor clinical outcome and that treating this anemia with RBC transfusions is associated with even worse clinical outcomes have led to a search for other alternatives to RBC transfusion to treat anemia in the critically ill [1]. This chapter will focus on the roles of iron therapy, erythropoiesis-stimulating agents (ESAs), and hemoglobin-based oxygen carriers (HBOCs) for the treatment of anemia in the critically ill.

9.2 Iron Supplementation

Iron studies in critically ill patients consistently demonstrate low iron and transferrin saturation with high serum ferritin levels; absolute iron deficiency is uncommon [7–9]. Many of these patients have a functional iron deficiency (FID) from redistribution of iron into macrophages and reticuloendothelial cells, limiting iron availability for erythropoiesis [3]. The fact that iron will promote bacterial growth has suggested from a teleological perspective that the low iron level observed in critical illness is a protective response to inhibit bacterial growth [3].

There are limited data available on iron supplementation in the critically ill. In a small trial in anemic ICU patients, intravenous (IV) iron supplementation failed to increase the reticulocyte count [10]. Similarly, neither oral nor IV iron was effective in either correcting anemia or reducing RBC transfusion in cardiac surgery patients [11]. In a study of enteral iron supplementation in critically ill surgical patients, there was a trend toward decreased RBC transfusion with iron supplementation in the subgroup of patients with evidence of FID as assessed by elevated erythrocyte zinc protoporphyrin (eZPP) [12].

Oral iron therapy, which even under the best of circumstances is poorly tolerated, may present a particular problem in the critically ill [13]. Hepcidin, a 25-amino acid hepatic peptide hormone, is an acute-phase reactant and the key regulator controlling intestinal iron absorption and distribution of iron from body stores. Hepcidin levels have been reported to rise to extremely high levels in critically ill trauma patients and are positively correlated with the duration of anemia [14]. High serum hepcidin levels decrease intestinal iron absorption as well as block iron export from tissue stores into the bloodstream. Therefore, absorption of oral iron in the critically ill may be limited. Recently, Pieracci et al. have reported the results of a randomized trial of IV iron supplementation (300 mg/week for 2 weeks) in critically ill trauma patients with anemia [15]. This study demonstrated that administration of IV iron alone was not sufficient to stimulate erythropoiesis in these critically ill patients. There was no positive effect of IV iron on FID, iron-deficient erythropoiesis, RBC transfusion, or clinical outcomes. However, eZPP levels were no different with iron therapy in the iron and placebo cohorts, suggesting persistent FID, and transferrin saturation achieved (16 %) was well below the ideal target for bone marrow iron delivery. Whether an alternative dosing strategy using higher doses of iron supplementation might be more effective remains unstudied. Overall, the data available to date provides little support for iron supplementation and supports the recommendation of the British Committee for Standards in Haematology that in the absence of clear evidence of iron deficiency, routine iron supplementation is not recommended during critical illness [16].

The major concern with iron therapy, particularly intravenously, has been the risk of infection. A recent meta-analysis of randomized trials of iron therapy in a range of patients found a significant increase in the risk of infection in patients who received IV iron compared with oral or no iron (RR 1.33, 95 % CI 1.110, 1.64) [17]. However, an increase in infection rate has not been observed in more critically ill patients. Torres et al. [18] found that in a cohort of 863 patients undergoing cardiac surgery, IV iron therapy was not associated with an increase in infection rate. Similarly, neither oral nor IV iron supplementation was associated with an increase in infections in critically ill trauma patients [12, 15].

The key role of hepcidin in AI raises the question of whether anti-hepcidin agents may have a role in the treatment of AI in critically ill patients. Several hepcidin antagonists are currently being tested in early clinical trials. The hepcidin inhibitor NOX-H94 (a structured mirror-image RNA oligonucleotide, Spiegelmer) is in a phase II trial to treat anemia associated with chronic disease [19]. A humanized antibody (LY2787106) that binds to hepcidin and neutralizes its function is being investigated in a phase I clinical trial in patients with cancer-associated anemia (NCT01340976). Finally, clinical trials are planned for Anticalin (a protein derived from human lipocalins) PRS-080 that specifically binds human hepcidin with subnanomolar affinity [20, 21]. The results of these clinical trials will help determine the future role of hepcidin antagonists as novel agents for the treatment of iron-restricted anemia.

9.3   Erythropoiesis-Stimulating Agents

A major feature of the anemia of critical illness is a failure of circulating erythropoietin concentrations to increase appropriately in response to the reduction in hemoglobin levels [7–9]. These observations have suggested that treatment with pharmacological doses of erythropoietin-stimulating agents (ESAs) might raise the hemoglobin concentration and as a result reduce allogeneic RBC transfusion requirements in critically ill patients. The rationale for ESA therapy is that increased erythropoiesis will result in higher hemoglobin levels, a more rapid return to normal hemoglobin levels, and thus a reduced need for RBC transfusions. A corollary to this is that by avoiding the negative effects of transfused RBCs, clinical outcomes would improve.

The above rationale almost two decades ago led to a small-randomized pilot study (160 patients) that demonstrated a significant reduction in the number of RBC units transfused in patients treated with epoetin alpha [22]. This was followed by a much larger multicenter randomized trial (1,302 patients) that confirmed the finding of RBC transfusion reduction [8]. Similarly, a small trial of patients in a long-term acute care setting demonstrated RBC transfusion reduction with epoetin alpha treatment [23]. However, a second large multicenter randomized trial (1,460 patients) found no RBC transfusion reduction with epoetin alpha treatment, although hemoglobin concentration did rise [9]. Importantly, in this latter trial, there was a significant increase in thrombotic events noted with epoetin alpha treatment. A meta-analysis of nine clinical trials, including the studies above, suggested a small reduction in RBC transfusion with ESA therapy [24]. The meta-analysis, however, was dominated by the two large trials that provided over 80 % of the patients analyzed [8, 9]. Conclusions regarding the safety and efficacy can thus be best drawn from these two trials.

Does epoetin alpha therapy decrease RBC transfusions? There appears to be no reduction in RBC transfusion with epoetin alpha therapy with recent more restrictive RBC transfusion practice [9]. The reduction in the percent of patients transfused and total RBC units transfused noted in the initial randomized trial [8] was not observed in the more recent trial [9]. The difference in results between the most recent trial and earlier trials results from a significant change in transfusion practice over intervening years. There was a significant increase in hemoglobin concentration with epoetin alpha therapy, demonstrating that epoetin alpha did have the expected hematopoietic effect, despite the absence of transfusion reduction. Epoetin alpha therapy in the critically ill appears to be associated with an increase in thrombotic events [9]. This is consistent with trials in non-critically ill populations (cancer and chronic renal failure) where epoetin alpha used to achieve higher target hemoglobin concentrations (i.e., above 12 g/dL) has shown an increased risk of thrombotic complications and mortality [25]. A post hoc analysis in the recent trial suggested that this risk might be mitigated by the use of prophylactic anticoagulation.

Does epoetin alpha therapy improve other clinical outcomes? Epoetin alpha appears to decrease mortality in trauma patients admitted to the ICU for greater than 48 h. This was suggested in a post hoc analysis in the initial large clinical trial [8] and confirmed in a prospective analysis in the most recent trial [9]. Taken together, the two trials, which included 1,433 trauma patients, provide strong evidence in support of a mortality benefit for epoetin alpha in trauma patients [26]. Functional outcomes in trauma patients receiving epoetin alpha for up to 12 weeks after hospital discharge were not improved [27]. In contrast to trauma patients, mortality was not significantly decreased in either medicine or surgery (non-trauma) patients receiving epoetin alpha – whether some subgroups within these populations may benefit requires further study. In view of the absence of RBC transfusion reduction, the mortality effect observed in trauma patients is likely a result of non-hematopoietic actions of erythropoietin.

Multiple tissues express erythropoietin and the erythropoietin receptor in response to stress which mediate local stress responses [28, 29]. Erythropoietin is a cytokine with antiapoptotic activity and has been demonstrated in preclinical and small clinical studies to protect cells from hypoxemia/ischemia. These "non-hematopoietic" activities of erythropoietin in protecting cells could be responsible for improved outcomes in the critically ill trauma patient. These effects of erythropoietin are locally mediated through tissue protector receptors and modulate the actions of proinflammatory cytokines [28, 29]. More recently, efforts are being made to develop non-hematopoietic, tissue-protecting erythropoietin derivatives that could potentially avoid adverse effects of erythropoietin therapy [28]. Recent clinical interest has centered on the potential role for ESA in neuro-injury and myocardial and renal injury [30]. Whether ESAs will have a role in the treatment of trauma patients admitted to the ICU awaits further study.

At this point, the following recommendations are supported by the available data. First, ESAs should not be used for RBC transfusion reduction for patients admitted to the ICU, particularly medicine and surgical non-trauma patients, unless they have an approved indication for ESAs. Treating critically ill patients with ESAs would expose them to potential risk with no identifiable benefit in either transfusion reduction (assuming conservative practice) or clinical outcome. Second, prophylactic anticoagulation should be considered for critically ill patients who receive epoetin alpha. Third, whether erythropoietin alpha should be considered for trauma patients in the ICU remains an open question. The strength of the subgroup findings across the two largest studies [8, 9] suggests a potential benefit of epoetin alpha treatment for trauma patients admitted to the ICU for more than 48 h and meeting the other study criteria. However, any recommendation for routine treatment of trauma patients in the ICU with epoetin alpha awaits a confirmatory clinical trial. Future studies should focus on the non-hematopoietic actions of ESAs and their derivatives in the critically ill. A better understanding of these mechanisms may help to identify other populations that could potentially benefit as well as the best timing and dosing for ESAs.

9.4   Hemoglobin-Based Oxygen Carriers (HBOCs)

HBOCs are oxygen carriers that use purified human, animal, or recombinant hemoglobin in a cell-free hemoglobin preparation [31]. They are infusible oxygen-carrying fluids that have long shelf lives, have no need for refrigeration or cross-matching, could be in abundant supply, and are ideal for treating hemorrhagic shock in remote settings where blood is not available. A number of HBOC products have been developed and undergone preclinical and clinical testing as oxygen carriers and

Table 9.1 HBOCs status as of 2014

Product class	Product	Company	Technology	Status
Cross-linked Hb	HemAssist (ααHb, DCLHb)	Baxter	Cross-linked Hb	Discontinued; safety; increased mortality
		US army	Cross-linked Hb	
	rHb 1.1	Somatogen	Recombinant Hb	Discontinued; safety; hypertension
	rHb 2.0	Baxter	Recombinant Hb	Discontinued; safety
Polymerized Hb	PolyHeme	Northfield Laboratories	Glutaraldehyde, pyridoxal Hb	Discontinued; safety
	HBOC-201 (Hemopure)	OPK Biotech	Glutaraldehyde bovine Hb	Discontinued, approved for use in South Africa
	Hemolink	Hemosol	Polymerized Hb	Discontinued; safety; myocardial infarction
Conjugated Hb	PHP	Apex Bioscience	PEG-human Hb	Discontinued
	PEG hemoglobin	Enzon	PEG-bovine Hb	Discontinued
	Hemospan/MP4	Sangart	PEG-human Hb	Discontinued; no efficacy
	Sanguinate	Prolong Pharmaceuticals	PEGylated carboxyhemoglobin bovine	Phase I

PHP pyridoxylated hemoglobin polyoxyethylene conjugate, *PEG* polyethylene glycol

blood substitutes, and some have been discontinued related to safety issues (Table 9.1) [32]. The HBOCs that have undergone phase III clinical trials have very different characteristics as compared to RBCs (Table 9.2). To date, only one product (Oxyglobin, polymerized bovine hemoglobin, OPK Biotech) is licensed for veterinary use, and only one product (Hemopure, polymerized bovine hemoglobin, OPK Biotech) is approved for limited use in humans in South Africa when blood is not available [33].

The "first-generation" HBOCs were based on observations that cross-linking overcame hemoglobin subunit dissociation and renal toxicity. Experience with these solutions has shown that they can be vasoactive, sometimes increasing blood pressure, sometimes decreasing tissue perfusion, and sometimes both. Clinical trials were disappointing because of toxicity. A first-generation HBOC diaspirin cross-linked Hb (DCLHb, HemAssist) circumvented the safety concerns from dimerization of the hemoglobin tetramer by cross-linking the alpha chains chemically. However, clinical studies performed with human cross-linked hemoglobin (DCLHb) were stopped because of an increased mortality in two clinical trials in patients who received DCLHb after stroke and multiple injuries [34, 35]. Additional studies in cardiac and noncardiac surgery documented additional safety concerns with early study termination related to serious adverse events [36–38].

Table 9.2 Characteristics of HBOCs studied in phase III trials compared to characteristics of RBCs

Characteristic	Hemopure	PolyHeme	Hemospan, MP4	RBCs
Source	Bovine Hb	Human Hb	Human Hb	Human
Volume, mL	250	500	250 or 500	250–300
Preparation	Ready to use	Ready to use	Ready to use	Testing, typing, cross-matching
Compatibility	Universal	Universal	Universal	Type specific
Storage	Room temperature	Room temperature	Room temperature	Refrigerated
Hemoglobin (g/dL)	13 g/dL	10 g/dL	4.2 g/dL	13 g/dL
Unit equivalent (g)	30 g	50 g	21 g (500)	50 g
Molecular weight (>64 kDa)	≥95 %	≥99 %	≥99 %	≥100 %
P_{50} (mmHg)	38	29	6	26
Oncotic pressure (mmHg)	25	23	50	25
Viscosity	1.3 cp	2.1 cp	2.5 cp	Whole blood = 5–10 cp
Methemoglobin (%)	<10	<8	<0.5	<1
Tetramer, %	≤3.0	≤1.0	0	N/A
Half-life	19 h	24 h	43 h	31 days
Shelf life at 4 °C	≥3 years	≥1.5 years	>1 year	42 days
Shelf life at 21 °C	≥2 years	≥6 weeks	>1 year	≥6 h

Hb hemoglobin, *Cp* centipoises, P_{50} tension when hemoglobin-binding sites are 50 % saturated

The "second-generation" HBOCs were based on a better understanding of the mechanisms of this vasoconstriction and specific modifications to reduce nitric oxide binding and resultant vasoconstriction. Hemopure is a polymerized bovine hemoglobin product with a p-50 of 30 mmHg that is closer to human hemoglobin than stroma-free hemoglobin. When infused, these linked hemoglobin molecules circulate in the plasma, are smaller, and have a lower viscosity and more readily release oxygen to tissues than allogeneic red blood cells [39]. A similar bovine hemoglobin substitute is used in veterinary medicine as Oxyglobin (HBOC-301), approved to treat canine anemia in 1998. Hemopure was approved for the treatment of perioperative acute anemia, with the intention of eliminating or reducing the need for allogeneic RBC transfusion, in elective adult surgical patients in South Africa in 2001. However, in the United States, phase III trials with Hemopure were put on hold due to safety issues. The main reason was the adverse effect profile of the compound, in particular an increase in the risk of stroke and myocardial infarction. Hemopure can be used for compassionate use for the treatment of severe anemia in Jehovah's Witness patients but requires patient consent, institutional review board approval, and FDA emergency IND approval for use in individual patients.

Sanguinate is a bovine PEGylated carboxyhemoglobin developed to combine the beneficial functions of a carbon monoxide-releasing molecule (to promote antiinflammatory and anti-vasoconstriction effects) with an oxygen transfer agent. A phase I safety study was recently completed, and no serious adverse events were reported. A phase Ib trial in sickle cell patients is currently underway, and multiple phase II clinical trials are in development, including one for treatment of vasoocclusive crisis. Sanguinate is also available for use under an expanded access emergency IND program (as with Hemopure above) for treatment of Jehovah's Witness patients with severe anemia.

PolyHeme is a first-generation pyridoxylated polymerized hemoglobin made from outdated human blood. It has a half-life of 24 h, a shelf life longer than 12 months when refrigerated, and a p-50 of 28–30 mmHg. PolyHeme is now no longer being produced and is not available for use. Multiple clinical trials were completed to test the safety and effectiveness of PolyHeme during resuscitation as well as both intraoperatively and postoperatively. In a phase II randomized trial, PolyHeme reduced the number of allogeneic RBC transfusions in acute trauma [40]. The US Multicenter PolyHeme Trauma Trial was the first trial in the United States of a HBOC in the prehospital setting that employed a waiver of informed consent. This was a 714-patient phase III trial in trauma patients randomized to receive either PolyHeme or standard of care at the time of injury [41]. There was no statistically significant mortality difference (day 1 and day 30) between the PolyHeme and control cohorts. Although there were more adverse events in the PolyHeme group, the benefit-to-risk ratio of PolyHeme was deemed favorable when blood is needed but not available [42]. PolyHeme failed to receive FDA regulatory approval.

Hemolink (hemoglobin raffimer) is a polymerized hemoglobin product manufactured from donated human blood and O-raffinose cross-linked to produce a polyHb. A phase III multicenter, double-blind clinical trial was performed to determine if intraoperative autologous donation (IAD) with 10 % pentastarch or with Hemolink immediately before cardiopulmonary bypass confers a reduction in blood transfusion compared with standard clinical practice in primary coronary bypass patients. Hemolink use was associated with significantly reduced number of allogeneic RBC units and non-RBC units administered and lower overall transfusion rates. The company elected to discontinue further development of Hemolink in 2004.

MP4/Hemospan is a PEG-conjugated human hemoglobin that underwent clinical trials in the United States and Europe [43]. To further increase the circulation time, hemoglobin can be linked to a macromolecule to increase its size. Human or bovine hemoglobin that is conjugated with polyethylene glycol (PEG) is protected from renal excretion. MP4 underwent evaluation in two pivotal phase III studies in Europe. One study (prevention trial) evaluated the ability of Hemospan to prevent acute hypotension in orthopedic surgery patients undergoing first-time hip replacement procedures under spinal anesthesia (NCT00421200). Although hypotensive episodes were significantly less in the MP4 group, more MP4 patients experienced adverse events, and no significant difference in the composite morbidity and ischemia outcome endpoints was identified [44]. The second study (treatment trial) evaluated the ability of MP4 to treat acute hypotension in orthopedic surgery patients undergoing first-time hip replacement procedures under spinal anesthesia (NCT00420277). Although the mean total duration of all hypotensive episodes was significantly shorter in the MP4 cohort compared to standard care, certain adverse events did occur more frequently in the MP4 group (nausea, bradycardia, hypertension, oliguria), and no difference in the composite morbidity and ischemia endpoints was identified [45]. A phase IIb study of MP4 in traumatic hemorrhagic shock patients (NCT01262196) aimed to evaluate the safety and efficacy of MP4 treatment in trauma patients suffering from lactic acidosis due to severe hemorrhagic shock. According to the annual report filed by the company with the SEC, MP4 did not achieve its primary endpoint, number of patients discharged and alive after 28 days as compared to normal standard of care treatment.

Recombinant human hemoglobin (rHb) is manufactured using *E. Coli* with recombinant technology that can be used to induce a variety of cell types to synthesize functional hemoglobin. Modifications of the hemoglobin molecular structure can alter the properties of the molecule, allowing researchers to create hemoglobins with improved functionality or enhanced safety. A major advantage of rHb is that it can be manufactured resulting in an unlimited supply. A modified recombinant human hemoglobin (rHb1.1, Optro) was under development during the 1990s. This product circumvented the safety concerns from dimerization of the hemoglobin tetramer by cross-linking the alpha chains through recombinant engineering with rHb1.1 [46]. rHb1.1 was a first-generation HBOC with a nitric oxide scavenging rate similar to that of native human hemoglobin. rHb2.0 was a second-generation HBOC, created via genetic manipulation of the distal heme pocket of both the alpha and beta subunits of hemoglobin leading to steric hindrance for nitric oxide entry with a nitric oxide scavenging rate 20- to 30-fold lower than rHb1.1 but maintenance of effective oxygen binding and release [47]. Preclinical animal studies were promising confirming decreased pulmonary hypertension, diminished capacity to scavenge nitric oxide, and lack of modulation of pulmonary vascular permeability [48–52]. Although rHb2.0 appeared promising, no clinical trials were performed and funding of this initiative was suspended.

A number of new advanced HBOCs are undergoing development [53]. A complete discussion of these is beyond the scope of this chapter. However, several interesting compounds deserve mention.

A human-derived pyridoxylated hemoglobin polyoxyethylene conjugate, which is polymerized with superoxide dismutase and catalase (PHP), was developed to reduce free-radical-mediated oxidative stress and scavenge excess nitric oxide in catecholamine-resistant septic shock [54]. A phase III multicenter randomized trial was initiated of PHP as a treatment to restore hemodynamic stability in patients with shock associated with systemic inflammatory response syndrome (SIRS). The study (NCT00021502) was terminated early due to difficulty with enrollment; however, analysis of the enrolled patients ($n = 62$) determined that PHP patients had quicker shock resolution, but the study was significantly underpowered for any meaningful analysis.

Cellular HBOCs consist of Hb molecules encapsulated inside oxygen carriers of different natures, aimed at mimicking red blood cell features. Cellular HBOC advantages consist of protecting the surrounding tissues and blood components from direct contact with potentially toxic tetrameric hemoglobin, avoiding the hemoglobin colloidal osmotic effect, prolongation of Hb circulation half-life, and not requiring the direct modification of the Hb molecule. With the application of nanotechnology, it is possible to achieve submicron-sized oxygen carrier and thus ensure oxygen availability to all body compartments. Two types of cellular HBOCs have been studied: liposome systems and polymeric microparticle/nanoparticle systems [55]. Liposomes appear to be retained in plasma for a significant period. By encapsulating hemoglobin with a stabilized phospholipid membrane, liquid-state preservation for 2 years is guaranteed at room temperature, and with dry powder, further prolonged preservation is possible. Modifying the method of preparing micro-dimension polymeric artificial cells can result in nano-dimension artificial cells. These nano-dimension artificial RBCs (80–150 nm in diameter) contain all the red blood cell enzymes. Recent studies show that using a polyethylene glycol-polylactide copolymer membrane, it is possible to increase the circulation time of these nano-dimension artificial red blood cells to double that of polyhemoglobin [56, 57].

RBCs can now be cultured in vitro from human hematopoietic, embryonic, or pluripotent stem cells, which represent a potentially unlimited source of RBCs. It also presents potential opportunities for development of a new generation of allogeneic transfusion products [58, 59].

Landmark studies showed that RBC obtained from an immortalized embryonic stem cell line can protect mice from lethal anemia [60] and that ten million RBCs (equivalent to 2 ml of blood) generated ex vivo from CD34 cells from an adult volunteer and transfused had in vivo survival comparable to that of native RBCs [61]. The recently established human-induced pluripotent stem (hiPS) cells represent potentially unlimited sources of donor-free RBCs for blood transfusion as they can proliferate indefinitely in vitro [62].

Adverse effects of HBOCs include hypertension, abdominal pain, skin rash, diarrhea, jaundice, hemoglobinuria, oliguria, fever, stroke, and laboratory anomalies such as an elevation in lipase levels. Although most of these side effects are transient and clinically asymptomatic, many clinical trials involving these agents have been discontinued or held due to the associated adverse effects. Current formulations appear to cause fewer severe effects compared to previous products; however, there remain concerns associated with HBOCs. It has been difficult to discern whether the adverse events that have been observed following the infusion of HBOCs in patients are related solely to the HBOCs or to other treatments administered to these patients during their routine care. A meta-analysis of 16 trials in adult patients ($n = 3,711$) involving 5 different HBOCs in varied patient populations reviewed data on death and myocardial infarction as outcome variables [63]. They reported a statistically significant increase in the risk of death (RR 1.30, 95 % CI 1.05–1.61) and the risk of MI (RR 2.71; 95 % CI 1.67–4.40). There are, however, many limitations to this analysis [64].

There remains an unmet need for HBOCs in a variety of medical situations, particularly in trauma and critical care. Despite the many HBOC products that have been developed and undergone preclinical and clinical testing at present, only one product (Oxyglobin, polymerized bovine hemoglobin, OPK Biotech) is licensed for veterinary use, and only one product (Hemopure, polymerized bovine hemoglobin, OPK Biotech) is approved for limited use in humans in South Africa when blood is not available. No HBOC is currently approved by the FDA for use in humans in the United States; however, Hemopure and Sanguinate are available for compassionate use in Jehovah's Witness patients with FDA EIND approval. There are now new approaches for modifying the intrinsic biologic properties of hemoglobin to produce improved HBOCs. The ultimate goal remains the availability of a safe HBOC for clinical use in the appropriate clinical situations.

9.5 Conclusion

Anemia is common in the critically ill; however, the treatment of this anemia with RBC transfusion is associated with an increase in risk but little evidence of clinical benefit in many clinical situations. However, alternatives to RBC transfusion for the treatment of anemia in the critically ill have been equally disappointing. At the present time, the following conclusions can be drawn: First, the data available to date provides little support for iron supplementation, and in the absence of evidence of iron deficiency, routine iron supplementation is not recommended during critical illness. The possible role of hepcidin antagonists as novel agents for the treatment of iron-restricted anemia awaits the results of future trial. Second, erythropoietin-stimulating agents should not be used for the treatment of anemia in the critically ill unless a patient has an approved indication for an ESA. For any critically ill patient who does receive an ESA, prophylactic anticoagulation should be considered. Any recommendation for the use of ESAs in trauma patients in the ICU must await further study. Future studies should focus on the non-hematopoietic actions of ESAs and their derivatives in the critically ill. Third, despite the many HBOC products that have been developed and undergone preclinical and clinical testing, at present there is no HBOC that has been approved by the FDA for use in humans in the United States. Only one product (Hemopure) is approved for limited use in humans in South Africa when blood is not available. New approaches for modifying the intrinsic biologic properties of hemoglobin to produce improved HBOCs may provide a therapeutic option in the future. At present the treatment of anemia in the critically ill should be guided by the fact that in the absence of acute hemorrhage, most critically ill patients tolerate a hemoglobin concentration in the 7 g/dL to 9 g/dl range and require no RBC transfusion.

References

1. Corwin HL, Gettinger A, Pearl RG, et al. The CRIT Study: Anemia and blood transfusion in the critically ill—current clinical practice in the United States. Crit Care Med. 2004;32:39–52.

2. Bateman AP, McArdle F, Walsh TS. Time course of anemia during six months follow up following intensive care discharge and factors associated with impaired recovery of erythropoiesis. Crit Care Med. 2009;37(6):1906–12.

3. Hayden SJ, Albert TJ, Watkins TR, Swenson ER. Anemia in critical illness. Am J Resp Crit Care Med. 2012;185:1049–57.

4. Carson JL, Carless PA, Hebert PC. Transfusion thresholds and other strategies for guiding allogeneic red blood cell transfusion. Cochrane Database Syst Rev. 2012;4:CD002042.

5. Marik PE, Corwin HL. Efficacy of RBC transfusion in the critically ill: a systematic review of the literature. Crit Care Med. 2008;36:2667–74.

6. Shander A, Gross I, Hill S, Javidroozi M, Sledge S. A new perspective on best transfusion practice. Blood Transfus. 2013;11:193–202.

7. Rodriguez RM, Corwin HL, Gettinger A, Corwin MJ, Gubler D, Pearl RG. Nutritional deficiencies and blunted erythropoietin response as causes of the anemia of critical illness. J Crit Care. 2001;16:36–41.

8. Corwin HL, Gettinger A, Rodriguez RM, et al. Efficacy of recombinant human erythropoietin in the critically ill patient: a randomized double blind placebo controlled trial. JAMA. 2002;288:2827–35.

9. Corwin HL, Gettinger A, Fabian T, May A, Pearl RG, Heard S, An R, Bowers P, Burton P, Klausner MA, Corwin MJ. Efficacy and safety of epoetin alpha in the critically ill. N Engl J Med. 2007;357:965–76.

10. van Iperen CE, Gaillard CAJM, Kraaijenhagen RJ, Braam BG, Marx JJM, van de Wiel A. Response of erythropoiesis and iron metabolism to recombinant human erythropoietin in intensive care unit patients. Crit Care Med. 2000;28:2772–8.

11. Garrido-Martin P, Nassar-Mansur MI, de la Llana-Ducros R, Virgos-Aller TM, Fortunez PMR, Avalos-Pinto R, Jimenez-Sosa A, Matinez-Sanz R. The effect of intravenous iron administration on perioperative anemia and transfusion requirements in patients undergoing elective cardiac surgery. Interact Cardiovasc Thorac Surg. 2012;15:1013–8.

12. Pieracci FM, Henderson P, Rodney JRM, Holena DN, Genisca A, Ip I, Benkert S, Hydo LJ, Eachempati SR, Shou J, Barie PS. Randomized, double-blind, placebo-controlled trial of effects of enteral iron supplementation on anemia and risk of infection during surgical critical illness. Surg Infect (Larchmt). 2009;10:9–19.

13. Goodnough LT, Nemeth E, Ganz T. Detection, evaluation, and management of iron-restricted erythropoiesis. Blood. 2010;116:4754–61.

14. Sihler KC, Raghavendran K, Westerman M, Ye W, Napolitano LM. Hepcidin in trauma: linking injury, inflammation, and anemia. J Trauma. 2010;69:831–7.

15. Pieracci FM, Stovall RT, Jaouen B, Rodil M, Cappa A, Burlew CC, Holena DN, Maier R, Berry S, Jurkovich J, Moore EE. A multicenter, randomized clinical trial of intravenous iron supplementation for anemia of traumatic critical illness. Crit Care Med. 2014. doi: 10.1097/CCM.0000000000000408.

16. Retter A, Wyncoll D, Pearse R, Carson D, McKechnie S, Stanworth S, Allard S, Thomas D, Walsh T, British Committee for Standards in Haematology. Guidelines on the management of anaemia and red cell transfusion in adult critically ill patients. Br J Haematol. 2013;160:445–64.

17. Litton E, Xiao J, Ho KM. Safety and efficacy of intravenous iron therapy in reducing requirement for allogeneic blood transfusion: systemic review and meta-analysis. BMJ. 2013;347:f4822. doi:10.1136/bmj.f4822.

18. Torres S, Kuo Y-H, Morris K, Neibert R, Holtz JB, Davis JM. Intravenous iron following cardiac surgery does not increase the infection rate. Surg Infect (Larchmt). 2006;7:361–6.

19. Schwoebel F, van Eijk LT, Zboralski D, Sell S, Buchner K, Maasch C, Purschke WG, Humphrey M, Zöllner S, Eulberg D, Morich F, Pickkers P, Klussmann S. The effects of the anti-hepcidin Spiegelmer NOX-H94 on inflammation-induced anemia in cynomolgus monkeys. Blood. 2013;121:2311–5.

20. Hohlbaum A, Gille H, Christian J, Allersdorfer A, Jaworski J, Burrows J, et al. Iron mobilization and pharmacodynamics marker measurements in non-human primates following administration of PRS-080, a novel and highly specific anti-hepcidin therapeutic [abstract]. Am J Hematol. 2013;5(88):E41.
21. Fung E, Nemeth E. Manipulation of the hepcidin pathway for therapeutic purposes. Haematologica. 2013;98:1667–76.
22. Corwin HL, Gettinger A, Rodriguez RM, Pearl RG, Enny C, Colton T, Corwin MJ. Efficacy of recombinant human erythropoietin in the critically ill patient: a randomized double blind placebo controlled trial. Crit Care Med. 1999;27:2346–50.
23. Silver M, Corwin MJ, Barzan A, Gettinger A, Corwin HL. Efficacy of recombinant human erythropoietin in the long term acute care patient: a randomized double blind placebo controlled trial. Crit Care Med. 2006;34:2310–6.
24. Zarychanski R, Turgeon AF, McIntyre L, Fergusson DA. Erythropoietin-receptor agonists in critically ill patients: a meta-analysis of randomized controlled trials. CMAJ. 2007;177:725–34.
25. Bohius J, Wilson J, Seidenfeld J, et al. Recombinant human erythropoietins and cancer patients: updated meta-analysis of 57 studies including 9353 patients. J Natl Cancer Inst. 2006;98:708–14.
26. Napolitano LM, Fabian TC, Kelly KM, Bailey JA, Block EF, Langholff W, Enny C, Corwin HL. Improved survival of critically ill trauma patients treated with recombinant human erythropoietin. J Trauma. 2008;65(2):285–99.
27. Luchette FA, Pasquale MD, Fabian TC, Langholff WK, Wolfson M. A randomized, double-blind, placebo-controlled study to assess the effect of recombinant human erythropoietin on functional outcomes in anemic, critically ill, trauma subjects: the long term trauma outcomes study. Am J Surg. 2012;203:508–16.
28. Brines M, Cerami A. Erythropoietin-mediated tissue protection: reducing collateral damage from primary injury response. J Intern Med. 2008;264:405–32.
29. Hand CC, Brines M. Promises and pitfalls in erythropoietin-mediated tissue protection: are nonerythropoietic derivatives a way forward. J Investig Med. 2011;59:1073–82.
30. Patel NSA, Nandra KK, Thiemermann C. Bench-to bedside review: erythropoietin and its derivatives as therapies in critical care. Crit Care. 2012;16:229.
31. Cabrales P, Intaglietta M. Blood substitutes: evolution from noncarrying to oxygen- and gas-carrying fluids. ASAIO J. 2013;59(4):337–54.
32. Jahr JS, Akha AS, Holtby RJ. Crosslinked, polymerized, and PEG-conjugated hemoglobin-based oxygen carriers: clinical safety and efficacy of recent and current products. Curr Drug Discov Technol. 2012;9(3):158–65.
33. Stowell CP. What happened to blood substitutes? Transfus Clin Biol. 2005;12:374–9.
34. Saxena R, Wihnhoud AD, Carton H, et al. Controlled safety study of a hemoglobin-based oxygen carrier, DCLHb, in acute ischemic stroke. Stroke. 1999;30:993–6.
35. Sloan EP, Koenigsberg M, Gens D, et al. Diaspirin cross-linked hemoglobin (DCLHb) in the treatment of severe traumatic hemorrhagic shock: a randomized controlled efficacy trial. JAMA. 1999;282:1857–64.
36. Schubert A, Przybelski RJ, Eidt JF, Perioperative Avoidance or Reduction of Transfusion Trial (PARTT) Study Group, et al. Diaspirin-crosslinked hemoglobin reduces blood transfusion in noncardiac surgery: a multicenter, randomized, controlled, double-blinded trial. Anesth Analg. 2003;97(2):323–32.
37. Lamy ML, Daily EK, Brichant JF, et al. Randomized trial of diaspirin cross-linked hemoglobin solution as an alternative to blood transfusion after cardiac surgery. The DCLHb Cardiac Surgery Trial Collaborative Group. Anesthesiology. 2000;92(3):646–56.
38. Schubert A, O'Hara Jr JF, Przybelski RJ, et al. Effect of diaspirin crosslinked hemoglobin (DCLHb HemAssist) during high blood loss surgery on selected indices of organ function. Artif Cells Blood Substit Immobil Biotechnol. 2002;30(4):259–83.

39. Cabrales P, Tsai AG, Intaglietta M. Balance between vasoconstriction and enhanced oxygen delivery. Transfusion. 2008;48(10):2087–95.
40. Gould SA, Moore EE, Hoyt DB, et al. The first randomized trial of human polymerized hemoglobin as a blood substitute in acute trauma and emergent surgery. J Am Coll Surg. 1998;187(2):113–20; discussion 120–2.
41. Moore EE, Moore FA, Fabian TC, Bernard AC, Fulda GJ, Hoyt DB, Duane TM, Weireter Jr LJ, Gomez GA, Cipolle MD, Rodman Jr GH, Malangoni MA, Hides GA, Omert LA, Gould SA, PolyHeme Study Group. Human polymerized hemoglobin for the treatment of hemorrhagic shock when blood is unavailable: the USA multicenter trial. J Am Coll Surg. 2009;208(1):1–13.
42. Moore EE, Johnson JL, Moore FA, Moore HB. The USA Multicenter Prehospital Hemoglobin-based Oxygen Carrier Resuscitation Trial: scientific rationale, study design, and results. Crit Care Clin. 2009;25(2):325–56.
43. Vandegriff KD, Malavalli A, Wooldridge J, Lohman J, Winslow RM. MP4, a new nonvasoactive PEG-Hb conjugate. Transfusion. 2003;43(4):509–16.
44. Olofsson CI, Gorecki AZ, Dirksen R, et al. Evaluation of MP4OX for prevention of perioperative hypotension in patients undergoing primary hip arthroplasty with spinal anesthesia: a randomized, double-blind, multicenter study. Anesthesiology. 2011;114:1048–63.
45. van der Linden P, Gazdzik TS, Jahoda D, et al. A double-blind, randomized, multicenter study of MP4OX for treatment of perioperative hypotension in patients undergoing primary hip arthroplasty under spinal anesthesia. Anesth Analg. 2011;112:759–73.
46. Burhop KE. The development of a second-generation, designer, recombinant hemoglobin. In: Artificial oxygen carrier, Keio University International Symposia for Life Sciences and Medicine, vol. 12. Tokyo: Springer; 2005.
47. Resta TC, Walker BR, Eichinger M, Doyle MP. Rate of NO scavenging alters effects of recombinant hemoglobin solutions on pulmonary vasoreactivity. J Appl Physiol. 2002;93:1327–36.
48. Malhotra AK, Kelly ME, Miller PR, et al. Resuscitation with a novel hemoglobin-based oxygen carrier in a Swine model of uncontrolled perioperative hemorrhage. J Trauma. 2003;54(5):915–24.
49. Fronticelli C, Koehler RC, Brinigar WS. Recombinant hemoglobins as artificial oxygen carriers. Artif Cells Blood Substit Immobil Biotechnol. 2007;35:45–52.
50. Hermann J, Corso C, Messmer KF. Resuscitation with recombinant hemoglobin rHb2.0 in a rodent model of hemorrhagic shock. Anesthesiology. 2007;107(2):273–80.
51. Raat NJ, Liu J, Doyle MP, et al. Effects of recombinant hemoglobin solutions rHb2.0 and rHb1.1 on blood pressure, intestinal blood flow and gut oxygenation in a rat model of hemorrhagic shock. J Lab Clin Med. 2005;145(1):21–32.
52. Von Dobschuetz E, Hutter J, Hoffmann T, Messmer K. Recombinant human hemoglobin with reduced nitric oxide scavenging capacity restores effectively pancreatic microcirculatory disorders in hemorrhagic shock. Anesthesiology. 2004;100(6):1484–90.
53. Kim HW, Greenburg AG. Toward 21st century blood component replacement therapeutics: artificial oxygen carriers, platelet substitutes, recombinant clotting factors and others. Artif Cells Blood Substit Immobil Biotechnol. 2006;34:537–50.
54. Chang TM. Blood substitutes based on nanobiotechnology. Trends Biotechnol. 2006;24(8):372–7.
55. Piras AM, Dessy A, Chiellini F, et al. Polymeric nanoparticles for hemoglobin-based oxygen carriers. Biochim Biophys Acta. 2008;1784(10):1454–61.
56. Chang TMS. Therapeutic applications of polymeric artificial cells. Nat Rev. 2005;4:221–35.
57. Baudin-Creuza V, Chauvierre C, Domingues E, Kiger L, Leclerc L, Vasseur C, Célier C, Marden MC. Octamers and nanoparticles as hemoglobin based blood substitutes. Biochim Biophys Acta. 2008;1784(10):1448–53.
58. Peyrard T, Bardiaux L, Krause C, Kobari L, Lapillonne H, Andreu G, Douay L. Banking of pluripotent adult stem cells as an unlimited source for red blood cell production: potential

applications for alloimmunized patients and rare blood challenges. Transfus Med Rev. 2011;25(3):206–16.

59. Zeuner A, Martelli F, Vaglio S, Federici G, Whitsett C, Migliaccio AR. Concise review: stem cell-derived erythrocytes as upcoming players in blood transfusion. Stem Cells. 2012;30(8):1587–96.

60. Hiroyama T, Miharada K, Sudo K, et al. Establishment of mouse embryonic stem cell-derived erythroid progenitor cell lines able to produce functional red blood cells. PLoS One. 2008;3:e1544.

61. Giarratana MC, Rouard H, Dumont A, et al. Proof of principle for transfusion of in vitro-generated red blood cells. Blood. 2011;118:5071–9.

62. Ebihara Y, Ma F, Tsuji K. Generation of red blood cells from human embryonic/induced pluripotent stem cells for blood transfusion. Int J Hematol. 2012;95(6):610–6.

63. Natanson C, Kern SJ, Lurie P, et al. Cell-free hemoglobin-based blood substitutes and risk of myocardial infarction and death. JAMA. 2008;299(19):2304–12.

64. Fergusson DA, McIntyre L. The future of clinical trials evaluating blood substitutes. Editorial. JAMA. 2008;299:2324–6.

Andrew Retter and Duncan Wyncoll

Abstract

Anaemia is extremely common in the critically ill and up to 50% of all patients admitted to critical care will receive a blood transfusion. No blood transfusion can be completely safe and there have been persistent concerns raised about possible increased mortality and morbidity associated with blood transfusion. These concerns prompted a number of studies examining restrictive transfusion practice. More recently, new devices have been developed to minimise blood loss associated with phlebotomy. This chapter will review the literature as regards specifically restrictive transfusion strategies. The later part will focus on therapeutic interventions, which can reduce the amount of blood lost to routine sampling. When a restrictive transfusion strategy is combined with the use of blood conservation devices, there is a trend towards a reduction in transfusion requirements. There is the potential to significantly reduce iatrogenic anaemia and consequently reduce the potential risk of any adverse consequences of transfusion.

10.1 Introduction

According to the SOAP study, 80 % of patients have a haemoglobin concentration of less than 90 g/L 7 days after admission to an intensive care unit (ICU) [1]. This study also examined both transfusion and phlebotomy practices, demonstrating a mean blood loss of 41 mL/day/patient due to phlebotomy. Equating to over 280 mL each week per patient, this volume is almost identical to that of a unit of red blood cells

A. Retter (✉) • D. Wyncoll (✉)
Department of Intensive Care, Guy's and St. Thomas' National Health Service Foundation Trust, London, UK
e-mail: duncan.wyncoll@gstt.nhs.uk

© Springer International Publishing Switzerland 2015
N.P. Juffermans, T.S. Walsh (eds.), *Transfusion in the Intensive Care Unit*,
DOI 10.1007/978-3-319-08735-1_10

(RBCs). In addition to phlebotomy, haemodilution and haemorrhage are the most significant contributors to the development of anaemia in the critically ill. The high rate of blood loss is compounded by impaired erythropoiesis secondary to inflammation, and high phlebotomy requirements impact increasingly with prolonged critical illness [2]. This extremely high prevalence of anaemia places a significant burden on the national blood services throughout the world with approximately 10 % of all RBCs transfused nationally given in general ICUs [3]. Of note, only about 20 % of these transfused RBCs are to patients who have active bleeding.

A number of publications have linked the transfusion of RBCs to potential harm in the critically ill. Although no definitive pathophysiological process has been proven, it has been demonstrated that blood transfusions are associated with an increased risk of infection and possibly mortality [4]. Despite the complex link between inflammation and the development of anaemia, it is rational to assume that if the volume of blood taken from a patient in routine testing can be reduced, then the development of anaemia may be slowed. This chapter reviews the more recent literature favouring restrictive transfusion policies in the ICU and discusses approaches to blood conservation.

10.2 Incidence of Anaemia and Frequency of Transfusion in Critical Care

Depending on case mix, between 30 and 50 % of patients receive an RBC transfusion during their ICU admission [2, 3, 5]. The majority of these transfusions are given to treat anaemia, with the mean blood volume administered ranging from 2 to 4 units per patient [1]. Despite substantial efforts to make blood safe, no transfusion is risk-free. In addition to the risks of transfusion-transmitted infection, ABO mismatch, volume overload and transfusion-related acute lung injury, the use of blood product support has been consistently associated with poorer patient outcomes.

In the European SOAP study, transfused patients had a longer ICU stay and higher associated ICU mortality [1]. This finding was corroborated by the North American CRIT study, which demonstrated that more transfused RBC units were independently associated with worse clinical outcomes and an admission haemoglobin concentration less than 90 g/L was also correlated with adverse outcomes [6]. These findings are supported by a recent systematic review of 45 studies focusing on patient outcome in relation to transfusion, where RBC use was found to be an independent risk factor for infection and the development of multi-organ failure [7].

10.3 Studies That Have Investigated Restrictive Transfusion Practice

The strongest evidence guiding transfusion policy in adult critically ill patients comes from the transfusion requirements in critical care (TRICC) study [8]. Patients with a haemoglobin concentration of less than 9 g/dL were assigned to one of two arms:

either a 'high' haemoglobin transfusion trigger of less than 10 g/dL with a target of 10–12 g/dL or a 'restrictive' target with a lower transfusion trigger with a haemoglobin concentration less than 7 g/dL. Mortality was compared at 30 and 60 days. The restrictive group received 54 % fewer units of blood with one third receiving no transfusion at all, whereas all the patients in the liberal group were transfused. The 30-day mortality in the liberal group was typical of general ICU populations, but there was a nonsignificant trend towards lower mortality for the restrictive group.

In two predefined subgroups, patients younger than 55 years and patients with an APACHE II score less than 20, the risk of death during the 30-day follow-up was significantly lower with the restrictive strategy. Patients aged less than 55 years who were enrolled in the restrictive arm had a 5.7 % mortality compared to 13.0 % amongst those in the liberal group. Similarly, patients with an APACHE II score less than 20 had an 8.7 % mortality versus 16.1 % when the restrictive and liberal arms were compared. These differences represented a number needed to treat to benefit from restrictive over liberal transfusion of about 13 for both these subgroups. Overall, there were also lower rates of new organ failures in the restrictive group and a trend towards higher rates of acute respiratory distress syndrome in the liberal group (7.7 % versus 11.4 %).

Despite the impressive results demonstrated in the TRICC study, persistent concerns have been raised about the applicability of the results to current practice. The possibility of selection bias has been raised as few patients with cardiac disease were enrolled and there was a high clinician refusal rate to allow randomisation. The study was also performed prior to the mandatory introduction of leucodepletion in many countries. Leucodepletion was introduced in an attempt to mitigate the risk of variant Creutzfeldt-Jakob disease infecting patients through the blood supply chain. Following this, there has been considerable debate as to the consequences of leucodepletion on the safety of blood. There has been a reduction in febrile nonhaemolytic transfusion reactions of around 60 %. CMV transmission has also been significantly reduced and there has been a decrease in the rate of HLA allo-immunisation [9]. The UK haemovigilance system has consistently shown a reduction in the incidence of transfusion-associated lung injury [10].

Despite the concerns of the TRICC study, the results have been supported by a number of other studies. The transfusion requirements after cardiac surgery (TRACS) study found no difference in a composite end point of 30-day mortality and severe comorbidity in cardiac patients prospectively randomised to a liberal or restrictive transfusion strategy [11].

The 'FOCUS' study, although not in critically ill patients, compared liberal with restrictive transfusion in high-risk patients undergoing hip surgery. There was no difference in mortality in the group assigned to the restrictive transfusion strategy [12]. It is important to emphasise that although patients in the FOCUS trial were not critically ill, they were elderly and had a high prevalence of cardiovascular disease.

To further study the use of 'restrictive' transfusion strategies in critically ill patients over the age of 55, Walsh and colleagues examined the outcome of critically ill patients ventilated for more than 4 days [13]. Patients were randomised to similar 'liberal' and 'restrictive' groups as previously defined. Baseline comorbidities and illness severity were high, and 32 % of patients had documented ischaemic heart disease. Mortality trended towards a higher rate in the liberal group, and no significant differences were observed in organ dysfunction or duration of ventilation.

A more recent study examined transfusion thresholds in patients with acute gastrointestinal bleeding. Villanueva and colleagues compared restrictive and liberal transfusion strategies in 921 patients [14]. Patients were randomly assigned, with 461 in the restrictive arm compared to 460 treated with a liberal transfusion approach. A total of 225 patients assigned to the restrictive approach as compared to 61 patients following the liberal pathway did not receive transfusion. There was also a reduced incidence of rebleeding, 10 % versus 16 % in the 'restrictive' arm. The probability of survival was greater at 6 weeks and the patients suffered fewer adverse events in the restrictive arm. However, when stratified into Child-Pugh score cirrhosis subgroups, there was no significant difference in patients with class C disease, probably reflecting the poor prognosis associated with severe advanced liver disease.

In summary, there is now an increasing body of literature that has studied restrictive transfusion practice with a consistent signal showing that 'restrictive' strategies reduce the amount of blood given to patients whilst revealing no clear detrimental effect.

10.4 Blood Sampling in the Critically Ill

Daily blood testing and arterial blood gas draws are the most common investigations performed in the critically ill. It is no surprise that the sickest patients require a higher frequency of blood sampling [15, 16]. Patients with arterial catheters have almost double the frequency of blood tests and a threefold increase in their volume of blood loss, and the total volume of diagnostic blood taken is an independent predictor of transfusion [17]. Arterial blood gases account for around 40 % of blood taken from ventilated patients [18].

10.5 Strategies to Optimise Blood Use in Critical Care

The general recommendations governing all transfusions remain applicable in the ICU. Clinicians should understand the indication for transfusion, specifically its potential risks and benefits. When possible, it is good practice to inform patients of the need for transfusion and obtain their consent. The indication for all transfusions should ideally be documented in the patient's notes. Basic investigations should always be completed to try to identify the cause of anaemia, and where an acceptable alternative to transfusion exists, this should be used in preference. Although relatively uncommon in the ICU population, examples include megaloblastic anaemia, microangiopathic anaemia, autoimmune haemolytic anaemia and iron deficiency anaemia.

There are several methods to reduce the volume of blood taken as part of routine testing. It is good practice to review phlebotomy requirement, particularly in those patients with ICU stays lasting more than 1 week. It is our experience that some patients can switch to alternate-day or even twice-weekly blood tests, particularly if they are stable. Maximum surgical blood ordering schedules (MSBOS), although predominantly aimed at improving laboratory productivity, promote the efficient use of blood. Their aim is to provide guidance to medical staff on the appropriate number of units to cross-match prior to a surgical procedure. This prevents inappropriate allocation of units, which may become out of date whilst they are assigned cross-match status. The introduction of MSBOS can have a significant and sustained impact to reduce unnecessary ordering of blood products without detracting from patient care [17].

10.6 Blood Conservation Devices

As previously mentioned, arterial lines are the most frequent port for blood sampling in the ICU. They are convenient and easy to access and when compared to central venous cannulas have a reduced incidence of line-associated infection. Conventional arterial line systems need an initial volume of 'deadspace' blood to be removed so that a sample of undiluted blood can be obtained for analysis. The initial draw is discarded, and given the frequency of testing, it becomes a significant contributor to accumulated daily loss. In normal use, the volume discarded is between 5 and 10 mL.

Blood conservation devices are based on a closed system, which enables the return of the deadspace portion of the sample. The device is attached to the patient's arterial catheter. A reservoir is used to siphon the blood into the reservoir for sampling; once collection is completed, a shut-off valve is opened and all the deadspace blood is returned through the arterial line to the patient. The blood conservation device is changed when an arterial line is replaced (typically every 3–4 days). The return of the otherwise discarded portion of the sample reduces the volume of blood lost, and there is evidence suggesting that this reduces the rate of anaemia in critically ill patients. Other potential advantages of blood conservation devices include a reduction in the incidence of line-associated infections, decreased sharp injuries and a reduced risk of accidental blood splash incidents.

10.7 The Evidence for Blood Conservation Devices

Studies have consistently demonstrated that blood conservation devices lead to a reduction in the volume of blood taken daily for phlebotomy. However, it has been difficult to show that they reduce the requirement for RBC transfusion [18–20]. The studies are all limited, as they are relatively small single-centre studies and none used a clear transfusion policy. To be most effective, a blood conservation device should be combined with a restrictive transfusion policy. This hypothesis has been tested in just a single study [19]. This trial examined the impact on transfusion requirements before and after the implementation of blood conservation devices. There was a slower rate of fall of haemoglobin levels between admission and discharge in the intervention group, and their use was independently associated with fewer transfusions of RBCs. Further analysis led the authors to suggest that blood conservation systems were of greatest benefit in patients with higher APACHE II scores, in patients receiving renal replacement therapy or in those who had a prolonged admission or were anaemic at admission to ICU [21].

Currently, there is no published data on the cost-effectiveness of blood conservation devices and it is difficult to quantify financial savings from the potential benefits of reduced transfusion, which may include a decreased length of stay and reduced mortality. However, anaemia is strongly associated with adverse patient outcomes and these devices do reduce the amount of blood taken from patients in routine testing. It seems prudent therefore that they should be adopted into routine practice. Indeed, evidence suggests that they have the greatest benefit in the sickest patients, who tend to have the longest hospital stay and are the most at risk of iatrogenic anaemia and the most likely to require blood transfusion.

10.8   Small Volume Blood Tubes

The use of paediatric blood tubes is an attractive and simple method allowing a reduction in daily phlebotomy volume. A small randomised controlled trial using a highly conservative phlebotomy protocol was performed by Harber and colleagues [22]. In this study the volume of each blood draw was recorded and the standard 5 mL of blood usually wasted after arterial blood gas sampling was returned. In the intervention group the median daily phlebotomy volume was 8 mL (range 7–10 mL) compared to 40 mL (range 28–43 mL) in controls. The study was limited as the median length of stay was short at 3 days, and as expected there was no significant difference in the rate of fall of haemoglobin. Despite clear advantages in terms of a reduction in iatrogenic blood loss, the study did not demonstrate a significant impact on the development of anaemia.

There are other significant limitations relating to the use of paediatric blood tubes. The cost of paediatric phlebotomy tubes is approximately three times greater than that of adult phlebotomy tubes, and the laboratory processing time is extended as the automatic blood analysers cannot 'handle' the tubes, which have to be processed by hand.

10.9   Conclusion

In conclusion, there are a small number of studies examining the use of blood conservation devices. Their advantages are appealing with a reduced risk of needlestick injuries and splashes to health care personnel, along with reduced blood wastage through routine phlebotomy. The literature consistently reports that patients lose less blood when these devices are used. However, they are only one part of good blood transfusion management [23]. There is a more substantial body of evidence to support the introduction of restrictive transfusion policies, and this is supported by many national guidelines [4]. When a restrictive transfusion strategy is combined with the use of blood conservation devices, there is a trend towards a reduction in transfusion requirements. There is the potential to significantly reduce iatrogenic anaemia and consequently reduce the potential risk of any adverse consequences of transfusion.

References

1. Vincent JL, Baron J-F, Reinhart K, Gattinoni L, Thijs L, Webb A, et al. Anemia and blood transfusion in critically ill patients. JAMA. 2002;288(12):1499–507.
2. Walsh TS, Saleh EE. Anaemia during critical illness. Br J Anaesth. 2006;97(3):278–91.
3. Walsh TS, Garrioch M, Maciver C, Lee RJ, MacKirdy F, McClelland DB, et al. Red cell requirements for intensive care units adhering to evidence-based transfusion guidelines. Transfusion. 2004;44(10):1405–11.
4. Retter A, Wyncoll D, Pearse R, Carson D, McKechnie S, Stanworth S, et al. Guidelines on the management of anaemia and red cell transfusion in adult critically ill patients. Br J Haematol. 2012;160:445–64.
5. Walsh TS, McArdle F, McLellan SA, Maciver C, Maginnis M, Prescott RJ, et al. Does the storage time of transfused red blood cells influence regional or global indexes of tissue oxygenation in anemic critically ill patients? Crit Care Med. 2004;32(2):364–71.
6. Corwin HL, Gettinger A, Pearl RG, Fink MP, Levy MM, Abraham E, et al. The CRIT Study: anemia and blood transfusion in the critically ill – current clinical practice in the United States. Crit Care Med. 2004;32(1):39–52.
7. Marik PE, Corwin HL. Efficacy of red blood cell transfusion in the critically ill: a systematic review of the literature. Crit Care Med. 2008;36(9):2667–74.
8. Hebert PC, Wells G, Blajchman MA, Marshall J, Martin C, Pagliarello G, et al. A multicenter, randomized, controlled clinical trial of transfusion requirements in critical care. Transfusion Requirements in Critical Care Investigators, Canadian Critical Care Trials Group. N Engl J Med. 1999;340(6):409–17. [Erratum appears in N Engl J Med. 1999;340(13):1056].
9. The provision of cytomegalovirus tested blood components. Position statement and more detailed report published March 2012 at: http://www.dh.gov.uk/health/2013/03/sabto/.
10. Report S. Serious hazards of transfusion. Annual report 2007. Serious hazards of transfusion scheme. 2008. http://www.shotuk.org.
11. Hajjar LA, Auler Junior JOC, Santos L, Galas F. Blood tranfusion in critically ill patients: state of the art. Clinics. 2007;62(4):507–24.
12. Carson JL, Carless PA, Hebert PC. Outcomes using lower vs higher hemoglobin thresholds for red blood cell transfusion. JAMA. 2013;309(1):83–4.
13. Walsh TS, Boyd JA, Watson D, Hope D, Lewis S, Krishan A, et al. Restrictive versus liberal transfusion strategies for older mechanically ventilated critically ill patients: a randomized pilot trial. Crit Care Med. 2013;41(10):2354–63.
14. Villanueva C, Colomo A, Bosch A, Concepcion M, Hernandez-Gea V, Aracil C, et al. Transfusion strategies for acute upper gastrointestinal bleeding. N Engl J Med. 2013;368(1):11–21.
15. Tarpey J, Lawler PG. Iatrogenic anaemia? A survey of venesection in patients in the intensive therapy unit. Anaesthesia. 1990;45(5):396–8.
16. Fowler RA, Berenson M. Blood conservation in the intensive care unit. Crit Care Med. 2003;31(12 Suppl):S715–20.
17. Richardson NG, Bradley WN, Donaldson DR, O'Shaughnessy DF. Maximum surgical blood ordering schedule in a district general hospital saves money and resources. Ann R Coll Surg Engl. 1998;80(4):262–5.
18. Thorpe S, Thomas AN. The use of a blood conservation pressure transducer system in critically ill patients. Anaesthesia. 2000;55(1):27–31.
19. Mahdy S, Khan EI, Attia M, O'Brien BP, Seigne P. Evaluation of a blood conservation strategy in the intensive care unit: a prospective, randomised study. Middle East J Anesthesiol. 2009;20(2):219–23.
20. Peruzzi WT, Parker MA, Lichtenthal PR, Cochran-Zull C, Toth B, Blake M. A clinical evaluation of a blood conservation device in medical intensive care unit patients. Crit Care Med. 1993;21(4):501–6.

21. Mukhopadhyay A, Yip HS, Prabhuswamy D, Chan YH, Phua J, Lim TK, et al. The use of a blood conservation device to reduce red blood cell transfusion requirements: a before and after study. Crit Care (London, England). 2010;14(1):R7.
22. Harber CR, Sosnowski KJ, Hegde RM. Highly conservative phlebotomy in adult intensive care – a prospective randomized controlled trial. Anaesth Intensive Care. 2006;34(4):434–7.
23. Page C, Retter A, Wyncoll D. Blood conservation devices in critical care: a narrative review. Ann Intensive Care. 2013;3(1):14.

Daniel Frith and Karim Brohi

Abstract

Transfusion in trauma has undergone a paradigm shift in the past decade. Previous resuscitation strategies for trauma haemorrhage featured early administration of large volumes of crystalloids with subsequent delivery of plasma to treat a gradually evolving coagulopathy due to haemodilution, hypothermia and acidosis. However, the identification of an acute endogenous coagulopathy in trauma victims triggered a re-evaluation of this strategy. Acute traumatic coagulopathy (ATC) occurs rapidly after severe injury as a product of combined tissue damage and hypoperfusion. A series of retrospective observational studies have identified that trauma patients receiving early (and high-dose) administration of haemostatic blood products (including plasma, fibrinogen and platelets), rather than crystalloids, may have better survival with reduced morbidity. This has been attributed to better prevention and/or treatment of ATC. Most western trauma centres now utilise a massive haemorrhage protocol to guide rapid delivery of these blood products in prespecified ratios. However, the re-emergence of thromboelastography is offering promise to refine this formulaic approach and replace it with patient-tailored algorithms. This chapter will describe the recent evolution in trauma transfusion with focus on our developing understanding of the coagulopathy driving these changes.

11.1 Introduction

The past decade has seen a paradigm shift in the mode of trauma-haemorrhage resuscitation. This was driven by the recognition of an acute traumatic coagulopathy (ATC) in severely injured victims and the potential for improved survival with

D. Frith, MBBS, MRCS, PhD (✉) • K. Brohi, FRCS, FRCA
Centre for Trauma Sciences, Queen Mary University of London, London, UK
e-mail: danfrith@me.com

© Springer International Publishing Switzerland 2015
N.P. Juffermans, T.S. Walsh (eds.), *Transfusion in the Intensive Care Unit*,
DOI 10.1007/978-3-319-08735-1_11

101

earlier administration of haemostatic blood products to treat it. This chapter will initially summarise the conventional concepts of traumatic coagulopathy, which have been understood and accepted for decades. They are generally iatrogenic in origin and develop gradually over time as a consequence of suboptimal resuscitation practices. It will then introduce and describe the aetiology and pathophysiology of ATC. This newly discovered entity develops rapidly after injury as a consequence of combined tissue disruption and systemic hypoperfusion. It is endogenous in origin and has led to a shift in our transfusion practices. These changes and potential future developments will then be discussed.

11.2 Conventional Concepts of Trauma-Induced Coagulopathy

Impairments of haemostasis after trauma result in difficult control of haemorrhage, increased transfusion requirements and worse mortality. Acute blood loss proceeds at a greater rate in the presence of systemic coagulopathy. Oozing of blood from blunt tissue injuries, vascular access sites and surgical incisions is not amenable to surgical control and may threaten viability. This uncontrollable haemorrhage may force the early termination of operations and result in the sacrifice of organs or limbs in order to preserve life. It also worsens outcomes from traumatic brain injury by an increased potential for intracranial haemorrhage and secondary neuronal damage.

Coagulopathy associated with trauma has been recognised for decades and is a constituent of the 'triad of death', together with hypothermia and acidosis. Classically it has been understood as due to loss, dilution or dysfunction of the coagulation proteases. Loss is explained as being due to bleeding or consumption, dilution from fluid administration and massive transfusion, whilst protease dysfunction results from hypothermia and the effect of acidosis on enzyme function.

Consumption of coagulation factors after trauma may not be limited to the location of tissue injury; trauma has frequently been cited as a disease that can precipitate disseminated intravascular coagulation (DIC). Whether trauma is a primary cause of DIC, as well as the mechanism through which DIC develops, is a matter of some scientific debate [1, 2]. Although systemic markers of coagulation activation (fibrin degradation products) are often elevated in trauma-induced coagulopathy (TIC), histological studies have failed to identify fibrin deposition, the hallmark of DIC. Whilst some bleeding trauma patients may be diagnosed and their prognosis categorised with DIC scoring systems, this is of limited clinical use because their specificity is poor and treatment is directed at the underlying pathology.

Until the most recent edition, the Advanced Trauma Life Support (ATLS) manual has recommended treating or preventing haemorrhagic shock by the initial administration of up to 2 l of crystalloid fluid. These synthetic products are capable of increasing intravascular volume and supporting tissue perfusion, at

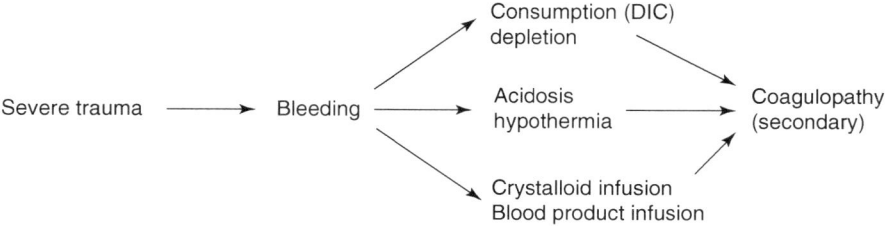

Fig. 11.1   The conventional concept of traumatic coagulopathy as a secondary process

least temporarily. However, they have no haemostatic content, and diluting residual circulating coagulation factors produces an iatrogenic coagulopathy in a dose-response fashion [3].

Mild hypothermia is very common in trauma patients and probably has minimal clinical impact. Contemporary studies of clinically important hypothermia (<35 °C) have reported an incidence rate of 1.5–8 %, and this is dependent upon the characteristics of the trauma cohort, their environment and the timing of the sample measurement [4–6]. The cause of hypothermia is multifactorial. From the time of injury, trauma itself alters the normal central thermoregulation and blocks the shivering response. Bleeding with subsequent systemic hypoperfusion creates an oxygen deficit and impairs heat-producing respiration, particularly in the large cutaneous and skeletal muscle beds. Trauma patients, who are frequently under the influence of alcohol, are then invariably immobilised with consequent loss of muscle activity and undressed to facilitate inspection and management of wounds.

Acidosis is a common event in trauma, typically produced by low-flow shock states and excess ionic chloride administered during resuscitation. When pH was reduced from 7.4 to 7.1 in pigs, Martini et al. showed that thrombin generation decreased to 47 % of control values, whilst fibrinogen concentration decreased by 18 % [7]. The depletion of fibrinogen was attributable to accelerated degradation rather than impaired synthesis [8]. These decreases were also associated with a 47 % increase in splenic bleeding time. Although acidosis can be corrected by the administration of buffer solutions, this does not correct the coagulopathy [9, 10], implying that the acid effect is more than simply a physical reduction in protease activity.

The traditional description of TIC depicts it as developing late after injury and as a consequence of continued haemorrhage and subsequent medical therapy. Figure 11.1 illustrates the putative unidirectional nature of this pathology. However, in the past decade, a series of research studies have demonstrated that some trauma patients arrive in the emergency department with a coagulopathy already established. These patients have generally had short transfers with little time to become hypothermic or receive significant exogenous fluid resuscitation. The impairment of their haemostatic system occurs early, develops endogenously and subsequently becomes exacerbated by the conventional causes of coagulopathy.

11.3 Acute Traumatic Coagulopathy

The first landmark report of the existence of acute traumatic coagulopathy (ATC) was in a retrospective study of the admission coagulation results of 1,088 trauma patients transferred to the Royal London Hospital by air ambulance [11]. Twenty-four per cent arrived in the emergency department with a clinically significant coagulopathy already established, and they were four times more likely to die than those presenting with normal clotting parameters. Subsequent studies performed by independent research groups on a total of over 45,000 patients have confirmed the existence of this early coagulopathy [12–17]. All of these studies reported a strong association between acute coagulopathy and mortality and identified it as an independent risk factor for death [12]. It has also been associated with longer intensive care and hospital stays. Patients are more likely to develop acute renal injury [15] and multiple organ failure [14] and have fewer ventilator-free days [13, 14], and there is a trend towards an increased incidence of acute lung injury [14].

Injury severity is closely associated with the degree of acute coagulopathy seen after trauma. In the London study, only 10.8 % of patients with an injury severity score (ISS) of 15 or below had a coagulopathy, compared with 33.1 % of those with an ISS over 15 [11]. This figure increased to 61.7 % for those with an ISS over 45. In a larger German study, a coagulopathy was evident in 26 % of patients with an ISS 16–24, in 42 % of patients with an ISS 25–49 and in 70 % of patients with an ISS > 50, respectively [14]. However, not all patients who are severely injured present with a coagulopathy; tissue trauma alone does not appear sufficient.

Shock with tissue hypoperfusion is a strong independent risk factor for poor outcomes in trauma [18, 19] and is central to the aetiology of ATC. One study of acute coagulopathy found that no patient with a normal base deficit (BD) had prolonged prothrombin time (PT) or activated partial thromboplastin time (aPTT), regardless of injury severity or the amount of thrombin generated [13]. In contrast, there was a dose-dependent prolongation of clotting times with increasing systemic hypoperfusion. Only 2 % of patients with a BD under 6 mmol/l had prolonged clotting times, compared with 20 % of patients with a BD over 6 mmol/l. The synergistic relationship between tissue injury, systemic hypoperfusion and severity of ATC has been characterised in an observational study of over 5,000 trauma patients [20] (Fig. 11.2).

Whilst it is accepted that tissue injury and systemic hypoperfusion are the principal aetiological drivers of ATC, the pathophysiology remains to be fully elucidated. Advocates of the DIC hypothesis propose that there is a rapid universal depletion of procoagulant factors caused by systemic consumption. However, contemporary evidence would indicate this is not the case. Functional activity of most coagulation factors required for thrombin activation is maintained at levels adequate for haemostasis. A few studies of *severely* injured trauma patients have identified a pronounced and isolated reduction of factor V down to activities around 30 %, a level consistent with prolongation of clotting times [21–23]. This might be of pathophysiological importance given that activated factor V is a target substrate for lysis by activated protein C. However, endogenous

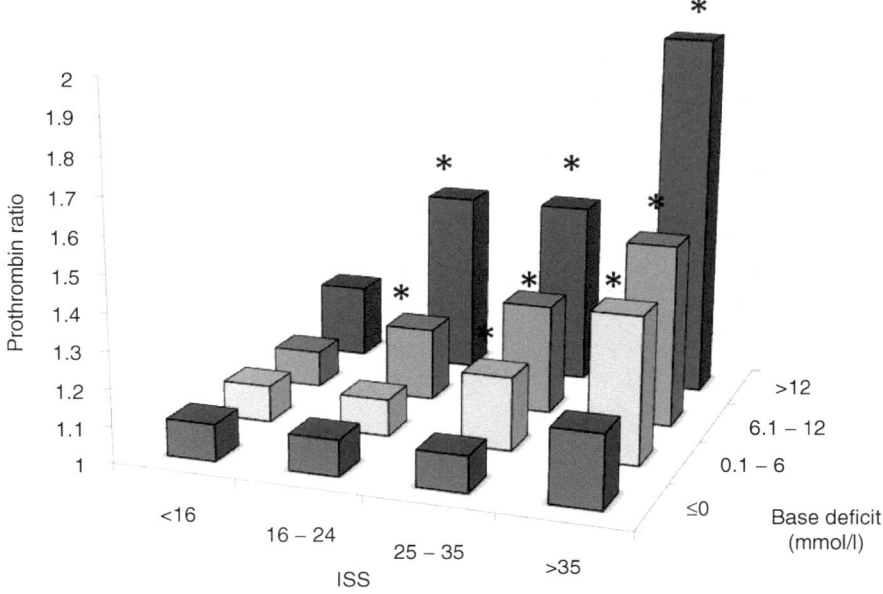

Fig. 11.2 The relationship between injury severity and shock. Mortality of patients grouped according to ISS and BD. *p<0.001 compared with ISS<16, BD ≤ 0 [20]

thrombin-generating potential has been reported to be normal or even enhanced in subjects with ATC [24].

Further downstream, clotting factor 1 (fibrinogen) is consistently reported as depleted early in trauma studies [25]. Concentrations below 1 g/dl acutely after injury have been reported, and thromboelastometric analysis frequently identifies an impairment of fibrin polymerisation. Unfortunately, at present, there are no rapidly available point of care tests available to measure circulating fibrinogen concentrations, and the optimal concentration necessary for effective haemostasis is unknown; contemporary guidelines recommend a plasma fibrinogen level of 1.5–2.0 g/dl [26].

Historically, TIC has been understood to develop exclusively in response to impairment or loss of procoagulant factors. The identification of ATC led to recognition of the pathological role of anticoagulant and fibrinolytic systems in response to trauma haemorrhage. Brohi et al. first identified a correlation between residual protein C depletion, assumed to be secondary to upregulated activation, and severity of ATC [13]. Subsequent clinical studies have confirmed the early activation of protein C after injury and its association with ATC, increased morbidity and mortality [23, 27, 28]. In a murine model, ATC could be blocked by inhibition of protein C activation using both pharmacological and gene-modulating methods [29]. Interventional clinical studies are required to determine the magnitude of influence this pathway, and other endogenous anticoagulants, has on ATC in humans.

Fibrinolysis is clearly a functional component of ATC. The impressive survival benefit associated with administration of tranexamic acid for traumatic haemorrhage highlights the pathological role of this pathway after injury [30]. Recent prospective clinical studies have better defined the incidence and clinical importance of this entity. Thromboelastometric analysis of 334 major trauma patients (ISS > 15) upon admission to the emergency room identified hyperfibrinolysis in 23, an incidence of 6.8 % [31]. In 14 cases, hyperfibrinolysis was considered fulminant with a complete breakdown of the clot observed within 60 min. A reduction of clot firmness between 16 and 35 % was observed in another nine patients. The mortality rate in patients with fulminant hyperfibrinolysis was 85.7 %, compared with 11.1 % in low-grade fibrinolysis. Patients with hyperfibrinolysis had higher ISS, lower Glasgow Coma Scale (GCS), lower systolic blood pressure and higher lactates than patients without hyperfibrinolysis. Amongst the majority of trauma victims that do not demonstrate hyperfibrinolysis on thromboelastometry, a significant proportion will experience 'occult' fibrinolysis with high D-dimers, which correlates strongly with poor outcomes [32].

Platelet counts are mildly reduced by trauma and this appears to associate with poor outcomes. A retrospective cohort study of 389 massively transfused trauma patients reported that in a logistic regression model controlling for ISS, GCS and admission BD, the odds of death at 24 h decreased by 12 % for every $50 \times 10^9/l$ increase in platelet count [33]. However, in most contemporary studies, they do not decline to levels that may be expected to contribute significantly to coagulopathy [27, 34]. Nevertheless, a few reports have identified that a high ratio of platelets to packed red blood cells is associated with improved outcomes [35]. This may lead us to conclude that the primary platelet impairment provoked by injury and/or haemorrhagic shock is functional. A study of 163 trauma patients has reported a minor, but significant, difference in platelet aggregometry parameters (ADTtest and TRAPtest) between survivors and non-survivors [36].

Vascular endothelium is an active participant in the pathophysiology of ATC. Large capillary beds host thrombomodulin and endothelial protein C receptors anchored through their luminal surface that capture thrombin and accelerate protein C activation 1,000-fold [37]. In addition to inactivating coagulation factors Va and VIIIa, aPC also consumes plasminogen activator inhibitor-1 (PAI-1), the major antagonist of tissue-type plasminogen activator tissue type plasminogen activator (t-PA). Consequently, traumatic haemorrhage with tissue hypoperfusion leads to overwhelming release of t-PA from vascular endothelial cells and subsequent hyperfibrinolysis [13].

Fascinating data is emerging, demonstrating an association between tissue hypoperfusion, neurohormonal activation and markers of endothelial disruption [38, 39]. In a prospective study of 75 adult trauma patients, circulating adrenaline levels were elevated in subjects with higher ISS, higher lactate and lower systolic blood pressure. This correlated positively and independently with the incidence of ATC as well as levels of syndecan-1, histone-complexed DNA, high-mobility group box 1, soluble thrombomodulin, t-PA and D-dimers. Trauma haemorrhage has been shown experimentally in rats to cause shedding of the endothelial glycocalyx.

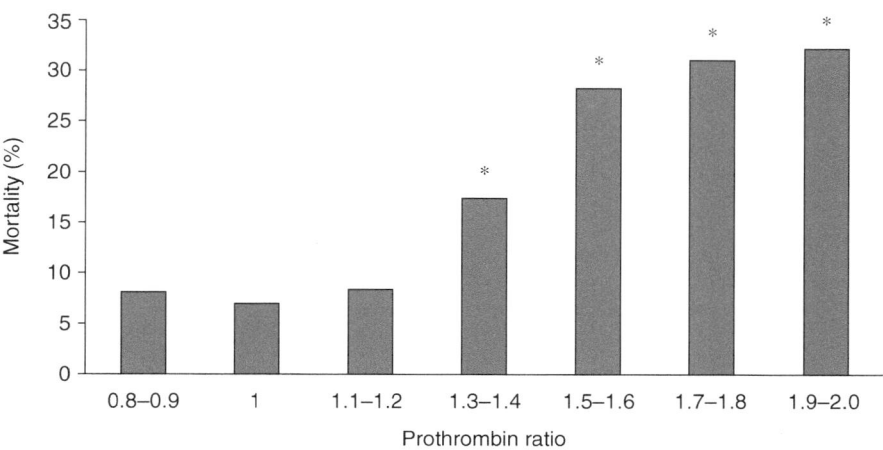

Fig. 11.3 The relationship between admission PTr and hospital mortality. $*p < 0.001$ compared with PTr = 1 [20]

Interestingly, this can be prevented by resuscitation with plasma, but not crystalloids or colloids [40]. Endothelial glycocalyx degradation is capable of triggering thrombin generation, protein C activation and hyperfibrinolysis. This is important because it indicates another potential mechanism by which tissue injury and shock mediate systemic anticoagulation early after injury.

11.4 Diagnosing TIC

Trauma-induced coagulopathy has conventionally been diagnosed as a prolongation of the international normalised ratio (INR) or aPTT greater than 1.5 times the normal value. However, the evidence for this diagnostic threshold is weak. More recently, the clinical relevance of different magnitudes of TIC has been elucidated (Figs. 11.3 and 11.4), and a prothrombin time ratio (PTr) or INR > 1.2 is now an accepted diagnostic definition of ATC [20].

Prothrombin time and aPTT are screening tests that report the time taken for initial fibrin polymerisation of platelet poor plasma, at 37 °C, in response to exogenous stimulation of coagulation. As such they neglect the pivotal role of platelets, do not measure clot strength and may not reflect haemostasis in vivo [41, 42]. Further, they are not reported expeditiously enough to accurately guide transfusion in the acute setting.

Recently there has been a renewed interest in the use of thromboelastometry for trauma care. These machines (ROTEM and TEG) employ a rotating pin or cup to measure the viscoelastic properties of ex vivo whole blood as it clots inside a small cuvette. They provide an assessment of the speed and strength of clot formation as well as fibrinolytic degradation over time. Research studies suggest their superiority

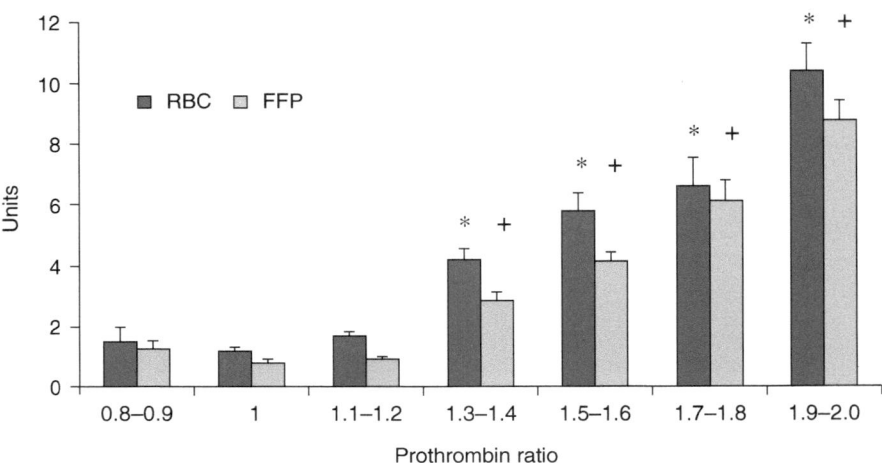

Fig. 11.4 The relationship between admission PTr and blood products transfused. *$p < 0.001$ compared with PTr = 1. +$p < 0.001$ compared with PTr = 1 [20]

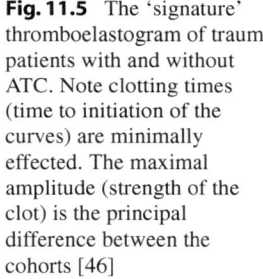

Fig. 11.5 The 'signature' thromboelastogram of trauma patients with and without ATC. Note clotting times (time to initiation of the curves) are minimally effected. The maximal amplitude (strength of the clot) is the principal difference between the cohorts [46]

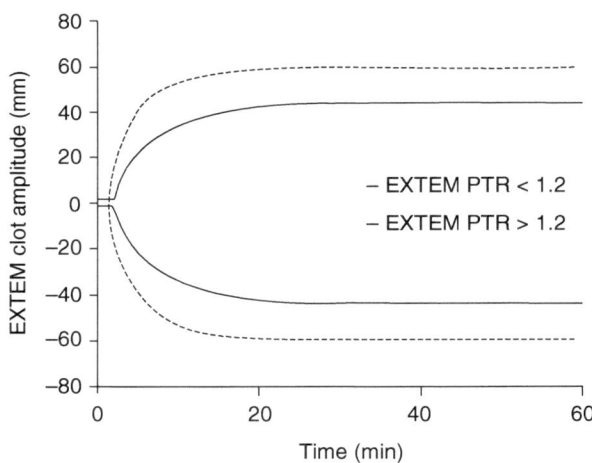

to routine tests of coagulation for diagnosing haemostatic impairments after injury [43, 44]. Trauma patients with ATC (defined as PT ratio >1.2) have a 'signature' thromboelastogram (Fig. 11.5). Compared to patients with PT ratio ≤1.2, the ATC trace is characterised by a reduction in clot strength with much smaller changes in clotting times and can be identified within 5 min – threshold of clot amplitude at 5 min (CA5) ≤35 mm (Fig. 11.6) [46]. Future studies using these machines will attempt to identify trace configurations associated with specific coagulopathy phenotypes. Further, they undoubtedly have a potential role in guiding transfusion in

Fig. 11.6 The clot strengths of patients with and without ATC can be reliably assessed at 5 min, rather than waiting for completion of the curve. This has significant advantages for rapidly directing tailored resuscitation [45, 46]

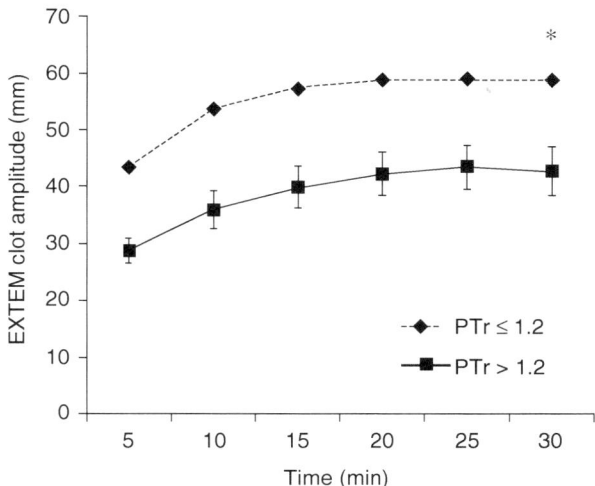

real time, and evidence-based treatment algorithms are required to determine our clinical responses to different trace patterns.

Although few patients with ATC demonstrate early depletion of platelets, monitoring the platelet count is useful to identify an emerging dilutional coagulopathy. However, these tests suffer from the same logistical problems as PT and aPTT tests and offer no assessment of platelet function. Platelet aggregometry is not widely available and is too slow to be of use in clinical care. Developments are occurring with viscoelastic tests to enable them to offer a point of care assessment of platelet responsiveness and contribution to clot strength. Given the increased use of platelet inhibitors within the population, this will be beneficial by helping clinicians tailor platelet therapy to individual patient haemostatic function rather than simple counts of platelet number.

11.5   Treating ATC

11.5.1 Conventional Treatment

Conventional trauma-haemorrhage transfusion protocols were developed during the latter half of the twentieth century to guide the delivery of different fractionated allogenic blood products. These guidelines most commonly recommended the administration of packed red blood cells to target a haemoglobin concentration of greater than 10 g/dl after trauma. Fresh frozen plasma (FFP) was not deemed required until the INR had exceeded 1.5 and platelets when their number dropped below 50,000 cells/mm³ [47–49]. Hence, it was not considered necessary to replace clotting factors until a dilutional coagulopathy was already established.

An increasing body of evidence developed to indicate that these protocols cannot and do not achieve normal haemostasis in trauma patients requiring a massive transfusion. A study from Houston examined the effectiveness of their pre-intensive care unit (ICU) massive transfusion protocol at correcting coagulopathy in severely injured and shocked trauma victims [50]. Ninety-seven patients receiving 10 or more units of packed red blood cells (PRBC) during hospital day 1 had a mean admission INR of 1.8 ± 0.2. Adherence to their massive transfusion protocol with administration of 5 units of FFP (commenced after the 6th unit of PRBC) together with 12 units of PRBC failed to correct this coagulopathy despite good management of hypothermia and acidosis. By the time of ICU admission 6.8 ± 0.3 h later, coagulopathy persisted (INR 1.6 ± 0.1), and this was identified as an independent predictor of mortality in this cohort.

11.5.2 Earlier and More FFP

During the first decade of the twenty-first century, data emerged from computer models and observational studies of trauma resuscitation protocols indicating that earlier and more aggressive treatment of coagulopathy with plasma and platelets could improve survival of trauma victims [3, 51]. A landmark retrospective study of the United States Army Joint Theater Trauma Registry analysed the effect of different plasma to red blood cell unit ratios on the mortality of trauma patients admitted to combat support hospitals in Iraq between November 2003 and September 2005 [52]. Two hundred and forty-six patients received 10 or more units of red blood cells (packed red blood cells or fresh whole blood), and they were grouped according to the ratio of plasma to red blood cells transfused. The low ratio group median was 1:8, the medium ratio group median was 1:2.5, and the high ratio group median was 1:1.4. Overall mortality rates were 65, 34 and 19 %, and haemorrhage mortality rates were 92.5, 78 and 37 %, respectively (Fig. 11.7). Upon logistic regression, plasma to red blood cell ratio was independently associated with survival (odds ratio 8.6; CI, 2.1–35.2).

This remarkable finding prompted clinicians to study their trauma databases to determine whether similar associations were present in the civilian sphere. Multiple retrospective reports flowed in the literature, mostly reporting a positive correlation between the ratio of FFP to PRBC delivered and survival. The first of these was a report by Duchesne et al. in 2008 from New Orleans, which divided 135 massively transfused trauma patients admitted between 2002 and 2006 into those that received a FFP to PRBC ratio of 1:1 and those that received a ratio 1:4 [53]. When the amount of PRBCs was greater than twice the number of units of FFP, a ratio of 1:4 was designated. A FFP:PRBC ratio of 1:1 was assigned to patients who received <2 units of PRBCs per unit of FFP given. Massive transfusion is associated with high mortality and 75 of the 135 cohorts (55.5 %) died. There was no difference in age, male gender, incidence of penetrating injuries, initial systolic pressure and ISS between the two cohorts. A significant difference in mortality was noted in patients with FFP:PRBC ratio of 1:4, 56 of 64 (87.5 %) versus 19 of 71(26 %), $p = 0.0001$. Patients in the 1:1 group died from ongoing bleeding, 3 of 19 (15.7 %) early after ICU admission within the first day and 16 of 19 (84.2 %) died of multiple organ failure at day 18 ± 12. In the

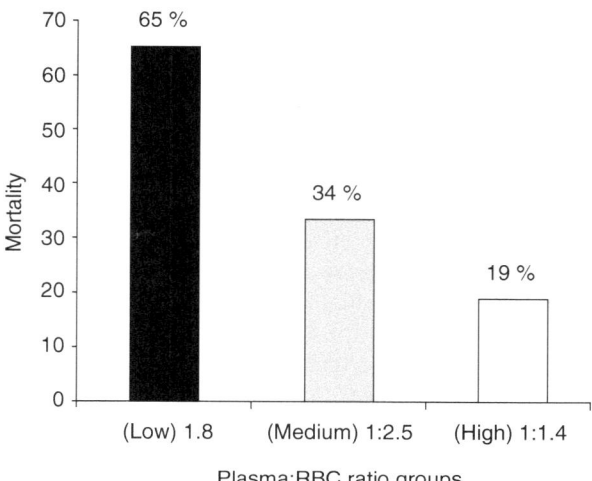

Fig. 11.7 The association between ratios of plasma received by injured soldiers during resuscitation and their risk of death [52]

1:4 group patients died from ongoing bleeding, 11 of 56 (19.6 %) early after ICU admission and 45 of 56 (80.3 %) died of multiple organ failure at day 16 ± 8. The authors noted that whilst their resuscitation practices addressed the 'acidosis' and 'hypothermia' components of the *lethal triad*, it neglected the third factor, coagulopathy. The title of their paper 'Review of current blood transfusions strategies in a mature level I trauma center: were we wrong for the last 60 years?' rightly questioned whether the practice of component blood therapy, which is logistically easier than delivering whole blood, was as clinically effective.

Most published studies originated from North American trauma centres, but a few similar reports emanated from Europe and Australia [54, 55]. Not all studies reported data consistent with improved survival from high-dose FFP. For example, a prospective study performed at the R Adams Cowley Shock Trauma Center in Baltimore selected 81 patients receiving a massive transfusion within 24 h (out of 806 trauma admissions) and calculated a logistic regression analysis to determine the effect of FFP:PRBC [56]. No significant effect on mortality was identified for either the PRBC to FFP ratio as a continuous variable (odds ratio (OR), 1.49; 95 % CI, 0.63–3.53; $p=0.37$) or 1:1 ratio as a binary variable (OR, 0.60; 95 % CI, 0.21–1.75; $p=0.35$) when controlling for age, gender, ISS, closed head injury, laparotomy status and ICU length of stay.

11.5.3 The Optimal Blood Product Ratio

There is a good potential rationale for administering high doses of plasma to patients receiving massive transfusion, as these are the subjects most likely to develop a dilutional coagulopathy. Reports of positive survival benefit with a high FFP:PRBC ratio in studies of non-massively transfused trauma patients are less numerous, perhaps because their procoagulant capacity never becomes diluted below a threshold necessary for satisfactory haemostasis. Further, results of some studies suggest that '1:1' resuscitation is unnecessary and a lower ratio, such as 2:3 or 1:2, could optimise haemostatic support whilst reducing harmful plasma side effects [45, 57]. Regardless, several meta-analyses performed on pooled data have concluded that a high ratio of FFP:PRBC is associated with a significant survival benefit for victims of trauma [58–60].

Prompted by these findings, several groups have performed similar studies looking at the effect of high platelet and/or fibrinogen administration and obtained broadly similar positive results [35, 61]. However, there is inherent survivorship bias in these observational studies that raises doubt on the validity of their conclusions. That is, fresh frozen plasma, which is the predominant source of plasma for most institutions, requires 30–45 min thawing and has conventionally been associated with a delay to administration compared with PRBCs. Therefore, patients with massive and ongoing haemorrhage often die during the early hours of hospital admission before receiving substantial quantities of FFP and thus are included in the low ratio cohort, whereas patients surviving long enough to receive sufficient FFP feature in the high ratio cohort. In other words, perhaps survivors receive plasma rather than plasma producing survivors.

Authors subsequently employed various strategies attempting to eliminate or minimise survivorship bias in their studies. For example, some only included patients who had survived the initial few hours when FFP administration typically lags. However, this strategy sometimes resulted in bias against FFP because early hospital death is frequently caused by rapid haemorrhage and this is the patient group who might be expected to benefit most from plasma. Another method used was to model the relationship between mortality and FFP:PRBC ratio over time and treat the ratio as a time-dependent covariate. Snyder et al. compared mortality of patients who had a high ratio at the end of 24 h with those who had a low ratio and found the former to be associated with increased survival [62]. This advantage became statistically insignificant when they divided the 24 h study period into 0.5–6 h subintervals and calculated the ratio and the mortality rates of both groups within each subinterval.

Obtaining a conclusive answer to the question of optimal blood product ratios to treat coagulopathy using observational studies alone is not possible. A multicentre, randomised trial (PROPPR – Pragmatic, Randomized Optimal Platelet and Plasma Ratios) will compare different ratios of blood products given to trauma patients who are predicted to require massive transfusions. Recruited subjects will receive blood products based on a 1:1:1 or 1:1:2 ratio of platelets, plasma and red blood cells. A total of 580 patients will be enrolled into this study from 12 participating sites in the United States and Canada, and it is estimated to report findings in 2015.

11.5.4 Massive Transfusion Protocols

Some investigators have hypothesised that earlier administration of coagulation delivers survival benefit rather than the precise ratio of products given. Delivering higher volumes of blood transfusion products to rapidly haemorrhaging trauma patients places significant logistical demands upon the local pathology service. Integrated 'massive transfusion' or 'major haemorrhage' protocols (MHP) have been developed to facilitate and direct the delivery of these products. Riskin et al. performed a 4-year cohort study to assess the impact of implementing MHP, aiming to deliver a FFP:PRBC ratio of 1:1.5 [63]. For the 2 years before and after MHP initiation, there were 4,223 and 4,414 trauma activations, respectively. The FFP:PRBC ratios were identical, at 1:1.8 and 1:1.8 ($p=0.97$). Despite no change in FFP:PRBC ratio, mortality decreased from 45 to 19 % ($p=0.02$). This was associated with a significant decrease in mean time to first product: cross-matched RBCs (115 to 71 min; $p=0.02$), FFP (254 to 169 min; $p=0.04$) and platelets (418–241 min; $p=0.01$). Effectively, catching up with coagulation support may not be as effective as preventing the impairment in the first place.

11.5.5 Other Haemostatic Agents

Whilst haemostatic resuscitation with a generic formula of blood products is the current practice in the United Kingdom and North America, it has not been implemented universally. Concerns regarding plasma transfusion-related side effects (e.g. immune-mediated adverse reactions, pathogen transmission, transfusion-related acute lung injury), better availability of coagulation factor concentrates and improved utilisation of point of care tests have combined to offer some European trauma centres an alternative, patient-tailored resuscitation solution. For example, in some Austrian centres, resuscitation commences with PRBCs and crystalloids. Recombinant fibrinogen concentrate is then given early to patients who demonstrate impaired fibrin polymerisation on their admission or subsequent viscoelastic test. Platelets are administered to subjects with continued clot weakness despite adequate fibrin function. Prothrombin complex concentrate (PCC, a mixture of recombinant vitamin K-dependent coagulation factors) is supplemented only to those who develop prolonged clotting times on viscoelastic testing (used as a surrogate measure of insufficient thrombin potential). Plasma is rarely indicated in this resuscitation protocol. Some retrospective cohort analyses have associated improved survival and reduced blood product use with this strategy [64].

Use of coagulation factor concentrates is logistically easier and targets specific defects in haemostasis. However, concentrates are expensive and their side-effect profile is not as well characterised as plasma. It is also not known whether focused replacement of coagulation factor deficits is more clinically effective than generalised support of the coagulation cascade. Finally, goal-directed management requires rapid results from validated tests of haemostasis using evidence-based algorithms. It is possible that point of care viscoelastic tests will be able to provide this service, but substantial further study is required before the next paradigm shift in trauma transfusion is adopted.

Whilst debate about optimal haemostatic resuscitation protocols is likely to persist for the foreseeable future, some clear and concise evidence regarding haemostatic adjuncts is now available. Firstly, recombinant factor VII appears to have no role in the resuscitation of haemorrhaging trauma victims after the early termination of the CONTROL trial of recombinant factor VII [65]. Although it had previously been shown to safely reduce blood loss from trauma in a Phase 2 trial, the Phase 3 trial was stopped prematurely after recruiting 573 of 1502 planned patients because the overall mortality was unexpectedly low and recombinant VII had no positive effect on survival [66]. Conversely, CRASH2 was a successful double-blind, prospective, randomised, placebo-controlled trial that enrolled 20, 211 adult trauma patients with or at risk of significant bleeding in 40 countries [30]. Patients were randomly given either a standard dose of tranexamic acid ($n = 10,060$) or matched placebo ($n = 10,067$) within 8 h of injury. All-cause mortality within 28 days was significantly reduced in the tranexamic acid group compared with the placebo group (risk ratio [RR] = 0.91; 95 % CI 0.85–0.97; $p = .004$). The risk of death caused by bleeding was also significantly reduced with tranexamic acid compared with placebo (RR = 0.85; 95 % CI 0.76–0.96; $p = .008$) and was particularly apparent for risk of death caused by bleeding on the day of randomisation (RR = 0.80; 95 % CI 0.68–0.93; $p = .004$). There was no increase in fatal vascular occlusive events or in deaths caused by multiorgan failure, head injury or others. Tranexamic acid is a cheap and easily administered medication. Research is ongoing in an attempt to refine the indication and patient population with greatest potential benefit from this drug. However, until better clinical efficacy is proven with improved inclusion/exclusion criteria, tranexamic acid should be administered as per the published clinical trial (bolus of 1 g within first 3 h of trauma, followed by continuous infusion of 1 g).

11.5.6 Blood Pressure Target

The principles of haemostatic resuscitation have recently been combined with a strategy of 'permissive hypotension' to create a modern concept termed 'damage control resuscitation' [67]. Permissive hypotension refers to resuscitation targeting a sub-physiological blood pressure in order to minimise haemorrhagic loss whilst maintaining adequate perfusion to essential organ beds. It is not a new concept; evidence of attempts to avoid 'popping the clot' is centuries old. However, it returned to scientific consciousness with the publication of a landmark (nonrandomised) trial conducted in 1994 that showed a statistically significant 8 % absolute reduction in mortality for hypotensive patients with penetrating torso trauma assigned to delayed (in the operating theatre) compared with prehospital or emergency room fluid resuscitation [68]. Two subsequent studies on trauma patients with blunt and/or penetrating injuries failed to confirm the clinical benefit of permissive hypotension [69, 70]. More recently, a prospective trial of 90 trauma patients in haemorrhagic shock randomised subjects to a minimum resuscitation target of 50 mmHg or 65 mmHg (mean arterial pressure). Although the authors could not demonstrate a survival difference for the two treatment strategies at day 30, 24 h postoperative death and coagulopathy were increased in the group with the higher target minimum pressure. One major drawback to this study was that no statistically significant difference between the actual mean arterial pressure was observed between the two groups for the duration of the study (64.4 mmHg vs. 68.5 mmHg, $p = 0.15$). Nevertheless, citing this evidence, current European guidelines recommend a target systolic blood pressure of 80–90 mmHg until major bleeding has been stopped in the initial phase following trauma without brain injury [26].

11.6 Summary

The discovery of ATC spurred significant leaps in our understanding of the haemostatic responses to injury and shock resuscitation. Acute traumatic coagulopathy is now recognised as a rapidly developing endogenous process that can be exacerbated by resuscitation with fluids devoid of coagulation factors. Conversely, potential for improved survival with reduced morbidity has been demonstrated by rapid administration of haemostatic blood products. The precise pathophysiology of ATC requires better characterisation, and this will direct the focus of our efforts to treat ATC. The haemostatic status of a trauma victim is constantly evolving in response to tissue damage, systemic hypoperfusion and medical attempts to support trauma. Future resuscitation paradigms will become more patient tailored and incorporate diagnostic tools that are capable of guiding therapy in a more responsive way.

References

1. Hess J, Brohi K, Dutton R, Hauser C, Holcomb J, Kluger Y, Mackway-Jones K, Parr M, Rizoli S, Yukioka T, Hoyt D, Bouillon B. The coagulopathy of trauma: a review of mechanisms. J Trauma. 2008;65(4):748–54.
2. Gando S. Acute coagulopathy of trauma shock and coagulopathy of trauma: a rebuttal. You are now going down the wrong path. J Trauma. 2009;67(2):381–3.
3. Hirshberg A, Dugas M, Banez E, Scott B, Wall MJ, Mattox K. Minimizing dilutional coagulopathy in exsanguinating hemorrhage: a computer simulation. J Trauma. 2003; 54(3):454–63.
4. Beekley A, Watts D. Combat trauma experience with the United States Army 102nd Forward Surgical Team in Afghanistan. Am J Surg. 2004;187(5):652–4.
5. Martin R, Kilgo P, Miller P, Hoth J, Meredith J, Chang M. Injury-associated hypothermia: an analysis of the 2004 National Trauma Data Bank. Shock. 2005;24(2):114–8.
6. Wang H, Callaway C, Peitzman A, Tisherman S. Admission hypothermia and outcome after major trauma. Crit Care Med. 2005;33(6):1296–301.
7. Martini W, Pusateri A, Uscilowicz J, Delgado A, Holcomb J. Independent contributions of hypothermia and acidosis to coagulopathy in swine. J Trauma. 2005;58(5):1002–9; discussion 1009–10.
8. Martini W, Holcomb J. Acidosis and coagulopathy: the differential effects on fibrinogen synthesis and breakdown in pigs. Ann Surg. 2007;246(5):831–5.
9. Martini W, Dubick M, Pusateri A, Park M, Ryan K, Holcomb J. Does bicarbonate correct coagulation function impaired by acidosis in swine? J Trauma. 2006;61(1):99–106.
10. Martini W, Dubick M, Wade C, Holcomb J. Evaluation of tris-hydroxymethylaminomethane on reversing coagulation abnormalities caused by acidosis in pigs. Crit Care Med. 2007;35(6):1568–74.
11. Brohi K, Singh J, Heron M, Coats T. Acute traumatic coagulopathy. J Trauma. 2003;54(6): 1127–30.

12. MacLeod J, Lynn M, McKenney M, Cohn S, Murtha M. Early coagulopathy predicts mortality in trauma. J Trauma. 2003;55(1):39–44.
13. Brohi K, Cohen M, Ganter M, Matthay M, Mackersie R, Pittet J. Acute traumatic coagulopathy: initiated by hypoperfusion: modulated through the protein C pathway? Ann Surg. 2007;245(5):812–8.
14. Maegele M, Lefering R, Yucel N, Tjardes T, Rixen D, Paffrath T, Simanski C, Neugebauer E, Bouillon B. Early coagulopathy in multiple injury: an analysis from the German Trauma Registry on 8724 patients. Injury. 2007;38(3):298–304.
15. Rugeri L, Levrat A, David J, Delecroix E, Floccard B, Gros A, Allaouchiche B, Negrier C. Diagnosis of early coagulation abnormalities in trauma patients by rotation thrombelastography. J Thromb Haemost. 2007;5(2):289–95.
16. Niles S, McLaughlin D, Perkins J, Wade C, Li Y, Spinella P, Holcomb J. Increased mortality associated with the early coagulopathy of trauma in combat casualties. J Trauma. 2008;64(6):1459–63; discussion 1463–5.
17. Hess J, Lindell A, Stansbury L, Dutton R, Scalea T. The prevalence of abnormal results of conventional coagulation tests on admission to a trauma center. Transfusion. 2009;49(1): 34–9.
18. Siegel J, Rivkind A, Dalal S, Goodarzi S. Early physiologic predictors of injury severity and death in blunt multiple trauma. Arch Surg. 1990;125(4):498–508.
19. Rutherford E, Morris JJ, Reed G, Hall K. Base deficit stratifies mortality and determines therapy. J Trauma. 1992;33(3):417–23.
20. Frith D, Goslings J, Gaarder C, Maegele M, Cohen M, Allard S, Johansson P, Stanworth S, Thiemermann C, Brohi K. Definition and drivers of acute traumatic coagulopathy: clinical and experimental investigations. J Thromb Haemost. 2010;8:1919–25.
21. Floccard B, Rugeri L, Faure A, Denis MS, Boyle EM, Peguet O, Levrat A, Guillaume C, Marcotte G, Vulliez A, Hautin E, David JS, Négrier C, Allaouchiche B. Early coagulopathy in trauma patients: an on-scene and hospital admission study. Injury. 2010;43:26–32.
22. Rizoli SB, Scarpelini S, Callum J, Nascimento B, Mann KG, Pinto R, Jansen J, Tien HC. Clotting factor deficiency in early trauma-associated coagulopathy. J Trauma. 2011;71(5 Suppl 1): S427–34.
23. Cohen MJ, Kutcher M, Redick B, Nelson M, Call M, Knudson MM, Schreiber MA, Bulger EM, Muskat P, Alarcon LH, Myers JG, Rahbar MH, Brasel KJ, Phelan HA, del Junco DJ, Fox EE, Wade CE, Holcomb JB, Cotton BA, Matijevic N, PROMMTT Study Group. Clinical and mechanistic drivers of acute traumatic coagulopathy. J Trauma Acute Care Surg. 2013;75(1 Suppl 1):S40–7.
24. Dunbar NM, Chandler WL. Thrombin generation in trauma patients. Transfusion. 2009;49(12): 2652–60.
25. Rourke C, Curry N, Khan S, Taylor R, Raza I, Davenport R, Stanworth S, Brohi K. Fibrinogen levels during trauma hemorrhage, response to replacement therapy, and association with patient outcomes. J Thromb Haemost. 2012;10(7):1342–51.
26. Spahn DR, Bouillon B, Cerny V, Coats TJ, Duranteau J, Fernández-Mondéjar E, Filipescu D, Hunt BJ, Komadina R, Nardi G, Neugebauer E, Ozier Y, Riddez L, Schultz A, Vincent JL, Rossaint R. Management of bleeding and coagulopathy following major trauma: an updated European guideline. Crit Care. 2013;17(2):R76.
27. Johansson PI, Sorensen AM, Perner A, Welling KL, Wanscher M, Larsen CF, Ostrowski SR. Disseminated intravascular coagulation or acute coagulopathy of trauma shock early after trauma? A prospective observational study. Crit Care. 2011;15(6):R272.
28. Cohen MJ, Call M, Nelson M, Calfee CS, Esmon CT, Brohi K, Pittet JF. Critical role of activated protein C in early coagulopathy and later organ failure, infection and death in trauma patients. Ann Surg. 2012;255(2):379–85.
29. Chesebro B, Rahn P, Carles M, Esmon C, Xu J, Brohi K, Frith D, Pittet J, Cohen M. Increase in activated protein C mediates acute traumatic coagulopathy in mice. Shock. 2009;32(6): 659–65.
30. Shakur H, Roberts I, Bautista R, Caballero J, Coats T, Dewan Y, El-Sayed H, Gogichaishvili T, Gupta S, Herrera J, Hunt B, Iribhogbe P, Izurieta M, Khamis H, Komolafe E, Marrero MA, Mejía-Mantilla J, Miranda J, Morales C, Olaomi O, Olldashi F, Perel P, Peto R, Ramana PV,

Ravi RR, Yutthakasemsunt S, CRASH-2 trial collaborators. Effects of tranexamic acid on death, vascular occlusive events, and blood transfusion in trauma patients with significant haemorrhage (CRASH-2): a randomised, placebo-controlled trial. Lancet. 2010;376(9734): 23–32.

31. Tauber H, Innerhofer P, Breitkopf R, Westermann I, Beer R, El Attal R, Strasak A, Mittermayr M. Prevalence and impact of abnormal ROTEM(R) assays in severe blunt trauma: results of the 'Diagnosis and Treatment of Trauma-Induced Coagulopathy (DIA-TRE-TIC) study'. Br J Anaesth. 2011;107(3):378–87.

32. Raza I, Davenport R, Rourke C, Platton S, Manson J, Spoors C, Khan S, De'Ath HD, Allard S, Hart DP, Pasi KJ, Hunt BJ, Stanworth S, MacCallum PK, Brohi K. The incidence and magnitude of fibrinolytic activation in trauma patients. J Thromb Haemost. 2013;11(2):307–14.

33. Brown LM, Call MS, Margaret Knudson M, Cohen MJ, Holcomb JB, Wade CE, Brasel KJ, Vercruysse G, MacLeod J, Dutton RP, Hess JR, Duchesne JC, McSwain NE, Muskat P, Johannigamn J, Cryer HM, Tillou A, Pittet JF, De Moya MA, Schreiber MA, Tieu B, Brundage S, Napolitano LM, Brunsvold M, Beilman G, Peitzman AB, Zenait MS, Sperry J, Alarcon L, Croce MA, Minei JP, Kozar R, Gonzalez EA, Stewart RM, Cohn SM, Mickalek JE, Bulger EM, Cotton BA, Nunez TC, Ivatury R, Meredith JW, Miller P, Pomper GJ, Marin B, Trauma Outcomes Group. A normal platelet count may not be enough: the impact of admission platelet count on mortality and transfusion in severely injured trauma patients. J Trauma. 2011;71(2 Suppl 3): S337–42.

34. Borgman MA, Spinella PC, Holcomb JB, Blackbourne LH, Wade CE, Lefering R, Bouillon B, Maegele M. The effect of FFP:RBC ratio on morbidity and mortality in trauma patients based on transfusion prediction score. Vox Sang. 2011;101(1):44–54.

35. Holcomb JB, Zarzabal LA, Michalek JE, Kozar RA, Spinella PC, Perkins JG, Matijevic N, Dong JF, Pati S, Wade CE, Cotton BA, Brasel KJ, Vercruysse GA, MacLeod JB, Dutton RP, Hess JR, Duchesne JC, McSwain NE, Muskat PC, Johannigamn JA, Cryer HM, Tillou A, Cohen MJ, Pittet JF, Knudson P, DeMoya MA, Schreiber MA, Tieu BH, Brundage SI, Napolitano LM, Brunsvold ME, Sihler KC, Beilman GJ, Peitzman AB, Zenati MS, Sperry JL, Alarcon LH, Croce MA, Minei JP, Steward RM, Cohn SM, Bulger EM, Nunez TC, Ivatury RR, Meredith JW, Miller PR, Pomper GJ, Marin B, Trauma Outcomes Group. Increased platelet:RBC ratios are associated with improved survival after massive transfusion. J Trauma. 2011;71(2 Suppl 3):S318–28.

36. Solomon C, Traintinger S, Ziegler B, Hanke A, Rahe-Meyer N, Voelckel W, Schöchl H. Platelet function following trauma. A Multiple Electrode Aggregometry study. Thromb Haemost. 2011;106(2):322–30.

37. Esmon C. The protein C pathway. Chest. 2003;124(3 Suppl):26S–32.

38. Johansson PI, Stensballe J, Rasmussen LS, Ostrowski SR. A high admission syndecan-1 level, a marker of endothelial glycocalyx degradation, is associated with inflammation, protein C depletion, fibrinolysis, and increased mortality in trauma patients. Ann Surg. 2011;254(2): 194–200.

39. Johansson PI, Stensballe J, Rasmussen LS, Ostrowski SR. High circulating adrenaline levels at admission predict increased mortality after trauma. J Trauma Acute Care Surg. 2012;72: 428–36.

40. Torres LN, Sondeen JL, Ji L, Dubick MA, Filho IT. Evaluation of resuscitation fluids on endothelial glycocalyx, venular blood flow, and coagulation function after hemorrhagic shock in rats. J Trauma Acute Care Surg. 2013;75(5):759–66.

41. Segal J, Dzik W, Transfusion Medicine/Hemostasis Clinical Trials Network. Paucity of studies to support that abnormal coagulation test results predict bleeding in the setting of invasive procedures: an evidence-based review. Transfusion. 2005;45(9):1413–25.

42. Levi M, Opal S. Coagulation abnormalities in critically ill patients. Crit Care. 2006;10(4):222.

43. Kheirabadi B, Crissey J, Deguzman R, Holcomb J. In vivo bleeding time and in vitro thrombelastography measurements are better indicators of dilutional hypothermic coagulopathy than prothrombin time. J Trauma. 2007;62(6):1352–9; discussion 1359–61.

44. Johansson P, Stissing T, Bochsen L, Ostrowski S. Thrombelastography and tromboelastometry in assessing coagulopathy in trauma. Scand J Trauma Resusc Emerg Med. 2009;17(1):45.

45. Davenport R, Curry N, Manson J, De'Ath H, Coates A, Rourke C, Pearse R, Stanworth S, Brohi K. Hemostatic effects of fresh frozen plasma may be maximal at red cell ratios of 1:2. J Trauma. 2011;70(1):90–5; discussion 95–6.

46. Davenport R, Manson J, De'ath H, Platton S, Coates A, Allard S, Hart D, Pearse R, Pasi KJ, Maccallum P, Stanworth S, Brohi K. Functional definition and characterization of acute traumatic coagulopathy. Crit Care Med. 2011;39(12):2652–8.

47. Lunberg, George D. Practice parameter for the use of fresh-frozen plasma, cryoprecipitate, and platelets. Fresh-Frozen Plasma, Cryoprecipitate, and Platelets Administration Practice Guidelines Development Task Force of the College of American Pathologists. JAMA. 1994;271:777–81.

48. O'Shaughnessy D, Atterbury C, Bolton Maggs P, Murphy M, Thomas D, Yates S, Williamson L, British Committee for Standards in Haematology, Blood Transfusion Task Force. Guidelines for the use of fresh frozen plasma, cryoprecipitate and cryosupernatant. Br J Haematol. 2004;126(1):11–28.

49. American Society of Anesthesiologists Task Force on Perioperative Blood Transfusion and Adjuvant Therapies. Practice guidelines for perioperative blood transfusion and adjuvant therapies: an updated report by the American Society of Anesthesiologists Task Force on Perioperative Blood Transfusion and Adjuvant Therapies. Anesthesiology. 2006;105(1):198–208.

50. Gonzalez E, Moore F, Holcomb J, Miller C, Kozar R, Todd S, Cocanour C, Balldin B, McKinley B. Fresh frozen plasma should be given earlier to patients requiring massive transfusion. J Trauma. 2007;62(1):112–9.

51. Ho A, Dion P, Cheng C, Karmakar M, Cheng G, Peng Z, Ng Y. A mathematical model for fresh frozen plasma transfusion strategies during major trauma resuscitation with ongoing hemorrhage. Can J Surg. 2005;48(6):470–8.

52. Borgman M, Spinella P, Perkins J, Grathwohl K, Repine T, Beekley A, Sebesta J, Jenkins D, Wade C, Holcomb J. The ratio of blood products transfused affects mortality in patients receiving massive transfusions at a combat support hospital. J Trauma. 2007;63(4):805–13.

53. Duchesne JC, Hunt JP, Wahl G, Marr AB, Wang YZ, Weintraub SE, Wright MJ, McSwain NE. Review of current blood transfusions strategies in a mature level I trauma center: were we wrong for the last 60 years? J Trauma. 2008;65(2):272–6; discussion 276–8.

54. Maegele M, Lefering R, Paffrath T, Tjardes T, Simanski C, Bouillon B, Working Group on Polytrauma of the German Society of Trauma Surgery (DGU). Red blood cell to plasma ratios transfused during massive transfusion are associated with mortality in severe multiple injury: a retrospective analysis from the Trauma Registry of the Deutsche Gesellschaft für Unfallchirurgie. Vox Sang. 2008;95(2):112–9.

55. Mitra B, Mori A, Cameron PA, Fitzgerald M, Paul E, Street A. Fresh frozen plasma (FFP) use during massive blood transfusion in trauma resuscitation. Injury. 2010;41(1):35–9.

56. Scalea TM, Bochicchio KM, Lumpkins K, Hess JR, Dutton R, Pyle A, Bochicchio GV. Early aggressive use of fresh frozen plasma does not improve outcome in critically injured trauma patients. Ann Surg. 2008;248(4):578–84.

57. Sperry JL, Ochoa JB, Gunn SR, Alarcon LH, Minei JP, Cuschieri J, Rosengart MR, Maier RV, Billiar TR, Peitzman AB, Moore EE, Inflammation the Host Response to Injury Investigators. An FFP:PRBC transfusion ratio >/=1:1.5 is associated with a lower risk of mortality after massive transfusion. J Trauma. 2008;65(5):986–93.

58. Murad MH, Stubbs JR, Gandhi MJ, Wang AT, Paul A, Erwin PJ, Montori VM, Roback JD. The effect of plasma transfusion on morbidity and mortality: a systematic review and meta-analysis. Transfusion. 2010;50(6):1370–83.

59. Johansson PI, Oliveri RS, Ostrowski SR. Hemostatic resuscitation with plasma and platelets in trauma. J Emerg Trauma Shock. 2012;5(2):120–5.

60. Bhangu A, Nepogodiev D, Doughty H, Bowley DM. Meta-analysis of plasma to red blood cell ratios and mortality in massive blood transfusions for trauma. Injury. 2013;44(12):1693–9.

61. Stinger HK, Spinella PC, Perkins JG, Grathwohl KW, Salinas J, Martini WZ, Hess JR, Dubick MA, Simon CD, Beekley AC, Wolf SE, Wade CE, Holcomb JB. The ratio of fibrinogen to red

cells transfused affects survival in casualties receiving massive transfusions at an army combat support hospital. J Trauma. 2008;64(2 Suppl):S79–85; discussion S85.

62. Snyder CW, Weinberg JA, McGwin G, Melton SM, George RL, Reiff DA, Cross JM, Hubbard-Brown J, Rue LW, Kerby JD. The relationship of blood product ratio to mortality: survival benefit or survival bias? J Trauma. 2009;66(2):358–62; discussion 362–4.

63. Riskin DJ, Tsai TC, Riskin L, Hernandez-Boussard T, Purtill M, Maggio PM, Spain DA, Brundage SI. Massive transfusion protocols: the role of aggressive resuscitation versus product ratio in mortality reduction. J Am Coll Surg. 2009;209(2):198–205.

64. Schöchl H, Nienaber U, Hofer G, Voelckel W, Jambor C, Scharbert G, Kozek-Langenecker S, Solomon C. Goal-directed coagulation management of major trauma patients using thromboelastometry (ROTEM)-guided administration of fibrinogen concentrate and prothrombin complex concentrate. Crit Care. 2010;14(2):R55.

65. Hauser C, Boffard K, Dutton R, Bernard G, Croce M, Holcomb J, Leppaniemi A, Parr M, Vincent J, Tortella B, Dimsits J, Bouillon B, CONTROL Study Group. Results of the CONTROL trial: efficacy and safety of recombinant activated factor VII in the management of refractory traumatic hemorrhage. J Trauma. 2010;69(3):489–500.

66. Boffard KD, Riou B, Warren B, Choong PI, Rizoli S, Rossaint R, Axelsen M, Kluger Y, NovoSeven Trauma Study Group. Recombinant factor VIIa as adjunctive therapy for bleeding control in severely injured trauma patients: two parallel randomized, placebo-controlled, double-blind clinical trials. J Trauma. 2005;59(1):8–15; discussion 15–8.

67. Holcomb JB, Jenkins D, Rhee P, Johannigman J, Mahoney P, Mehta S, Cox ED, Gehrke MJ, Beilman GJ, Schreiber M, Flaherty SF, Grathwohl KW, Spinella PC, Perkins JG, Beekley AC, McMullin NR, Park MS, Gonzalez EA, Wade CE, Dubick MA, Schwab CW, Moore FA, Champion HR, Hoyt DB, Hess JR. Damage control resuscitation: directly addressing the early coagulopathy of trauma. J Trauma. 2007;62(2):307–10.

68. Bickell WH, Wall MJ, Pepe PE, Martin RR, Ginger VF, Allen MK, Mattox KL. Immediate versus delayed fluid resuscitation for hypotensive patients with penetrating torso injuries. N Engl J Med. 1994;331(17):1105–9.

69. Turner J, Nicholl J, Webber L, Cox H, Dixon S, Yates D. A randomised controlled trial of prehospital intravenous fluid replacement therapy in serious trauma. Health Technol Assess. 2000;4(31):1–57.

70. Dutton RP, Mackenzie CF, Scalea TM. Hypotensive resuscitation during active hemorrhage: impact on in-hospital mortality. J Trauma. 2002;52(6):1141–6.

Vipul Jairath

Abstract

Acute upper gastrointestinal bleeding (AUGIB) is a common medical emergency which can present with life-threatening bleeding which is the single leading indication for transfusion of red blood cells in the UK. AUGIB is a condition associated with increasing age and comorbidity and with liver cirrhosis. Variceal bleeding in patients with liver cirrhosis presents a particular challenge due to multifactorial underlying derangements in coagulation, as well as the risks of exacerbation of portal hypertensive bleeding through injudicious volume replacement. A single high-quality trial has demonstrated that a restrictive approach to red blood cell transfusion (transfusion threshold of 7 g/dL) leads to a reduction in mortality and rebleeding, compared to a liberal transfusion strategy (transfusion threshold of 9 g/dL). However, this treatment effect was only significant for patients with liver cirrhosis, and the results cannot be generalised to patients with cardiovascular comorbidities. Although consensus guidelines recommend platelet transfusions to actively bleeding patients with a count of $<50 \times 10^9$, there is no evidence base to these recommendations, and this cannot be routinely advocated for AUGIB until there is further evidence. Similarly there is little evidence to guide plasma transfusion, and the harms associated with this intervention must be considered prior to transfusion. The presence of coagulopathy is associated with an increased risk of mortality, but it is unclear if this is simply a biomarker of illness rather than an indication for correction. Trials of antifibrinolytics have been shown to reduce mortality after AUGIB, but many of these studies were conducted before the advent of modern day endoscopy, raising uncertainty as to their effectiveness. Massive transfusion protocols should be used with caution in AUGIB due to the risk of volume overload in elderly patients. AUGIB is an

V. Jairath, BSc, MBChB(hons), DPhil, MRCP
Translational Gastroenterology Unit, Nuffield Department of Medicine,
University of Oxford, Oxford, UK
e-mail: vipul.jairath@nhsbt.nhs.uk

© Springer International Publishing Switzerland 2015   121
N.P. Juffermans, T.S. Walsh (eds.), *Transfusion in the Intensive Care Unit*,
DOI 10.1007/978-3-319-08735-1_12

important cause of morbidity and mortality worldwide and a major user group of all blood components, and therefore further research is justified to improve the evidence base for the approach to transfusion.

12.1   Introduction and Overview of Gastrointestinal Bleeding

Over the past decade, there has been considerable interest in optimising transfusion strategies in patients with trauma and major haemorrhage. In civilian hospital practice, however, gastrointestinal bleeding is the commonest acute medical emergency which can present with life-threatening bleeding and is an important cause of morbidity and mortality in high-, middle- and low-income countries. Of importance to agencies responsible for national blood supplies, digestive and liver diseases as a mixed case group are the commonest indication for transfusion of red blood cells (RBCs), fresh frozen plasma (FFP) and platelets in England [1]. Within this cohort, gastrointestinal bleeding is the single leading indication for RBCs, accounting for 12–14 % of all red blood cell (RBC) transfusions in England [2].

By convention, gastrointestinal bleeding is considered to either arise from the upper or lower gastrointestinal tract, arbitrarily defined as arising from either proximal or distal to the ligament of Treitz, respectively. Acute upper gastrointestinal bleeding (AUGIB) is more common with a UK annual incidence of 100–180/10, accounting for over 70,000 admissions annually [3], and can be broadly considered as non-variceal or variceal in origin. In western populations, non-variceal upper gastrointestinal bleeding (NVUGIB) accounts for over 80 % of AUGIB presentations, the major causative lesion being peptic ulcer disease (in 30–50 % of cases), followed by erosive disease. Risk factors include use of antiplatelet and non-steroidal anti-inflammatory drugs (NSAIDs), *Helicobacter pylori* infection, increasing age and comorbid illness. Acute variceal haemorrhage (AVH) in patients with liver cirrhosis accounts for approximately 10–20 % of presentations of UK presentations with AUGIB and is rising, largely driven by the increasing burden of alcohol and obesity-induced liver disease, and represents a particular challenge due to the severity of bleeding and complex underlying coagulation derangements in liver cirrhosis.

Lower gastrointestinal bleeding has an annual UK incidence of 20–30 cases per 100,000, the major causative lesions being diverticulosis, angiodysplasia, colitis, neoplasm and anorectal disease. Age is the major risk factor associated with lower GI bleeding (reflecting the higher incidence of conditions that tend to occur) as is use of NSAIDs and aspirin which cause mucosal injury throughout the GI tract. In Europe the incidence of lower GI bleeding is rising and of upper GI bleeding is falling, the latter probably due to decreasing incidence of helicobacter pylori infection [4].

Despite improvements in the outcomes of patients with AUGIB in the past two decades, mortality remains appreciably high, even in the most modern of healthcare systems [5]. In a recent nationwide UK audit, the case fatality for new presentations to the hospital was 7 %, rising to over 26 % in patients already hospitalised for another condition [6, 7]. Whilst this is likely to largely reflect the burden of comorbidity in patients with this condition, death directly due to haemorrhage is still estimated to account for approximately 20 % of deaths following AUGIB [8]. Rebleeding is a specific challenge in the management of AUGIB, occurring in up to 16 % cases of non-variceal and in 25 % of variceal bleeding, and is a strong predictor of mortality. Of particular interest is that rebleeding rates, which are arguably the best measure of interventions directly targeted at arresting bleeding, have not improved much over the past 15 years [5]. Patients with lower GI bleeding tend to present with less severe haemorrhage, require fewer transfusions and have reported case fatality in the order of 3–5 %. There are few data characterising the epidemiology, use of blood components and outcomes of patients with lower GI bleeding, and it will not be discussed further in this chapter.

Regardless of the source of bleeding with the GI tract, the principles of management of gastrointestinal bleeding are identical to any other major haemorrhagic process, including the need for timely and adequate resuscitation followed by definitive therapies to arrest bleeding, which include therapeutic endoscopy in the mainstay, but occasionally surgical or radiological intervention where there is failure to control bleeding. This chapter focuses on transfusion strategies for AUGIB. This includes a review of the coagulopathy of liver disease and reviews the evidence for the approach to transfusion in patients with liver cirrhosis and variceal bleeding, since this represents a group with complex derangements of coagulation, typically more severe haemorrhage and more likely to be managed on an intensive care unit, although reference is also made to other causes of AUGIB throughout. There is particular focus on the evidence base for the use of red blood cells (RBCs) as well as the use of adjunctive pharmacological strategies such as antifibrinolytics which also have potential to prevent rebleeding.

12.2   Liver Cirrhosis and Acute Variceal Haemorrhage

Liver cirrhosis is a major cause of morbidity accounting for 800,000 deaths annually worldwide [9]. In the UK, the incidence and prevalence is rising, with an estimated 8,000 new cases per year [10]. Gastroesophageal varices develop in half of patients with cirrhosis (40 and 60 % of compensated and decompensated cirrhotic patients) [11] with bleeding occurring at a rate of 5–15 % per year [12]. Varices form as a result of portal hypertension and are assessed by hepatic venous pressure gradient (HVPG). HVPG greater than 10, 12 or 20 mmHg are associated with the primary development of varices, variceal bleeding and continued bleeding/rebleeding, respectively, which is of particular importance when considering the approach to volume repletion and transfusion volumes following haemorrhage [13]. Each episode of variceal bleeding is associated with a 20–30 % mortality, with a 70 % risk of recurrent bleeding within 12 months. Although variceal bleeding is considered to be mainly due to the interplay of portal hypertension, local vessel wall abnormalities and endothelial dysfunction, the contribution of deranged haemostasis as a precipitant of bleeding or as an aggravating factor during bleeding is poorly understood [14].

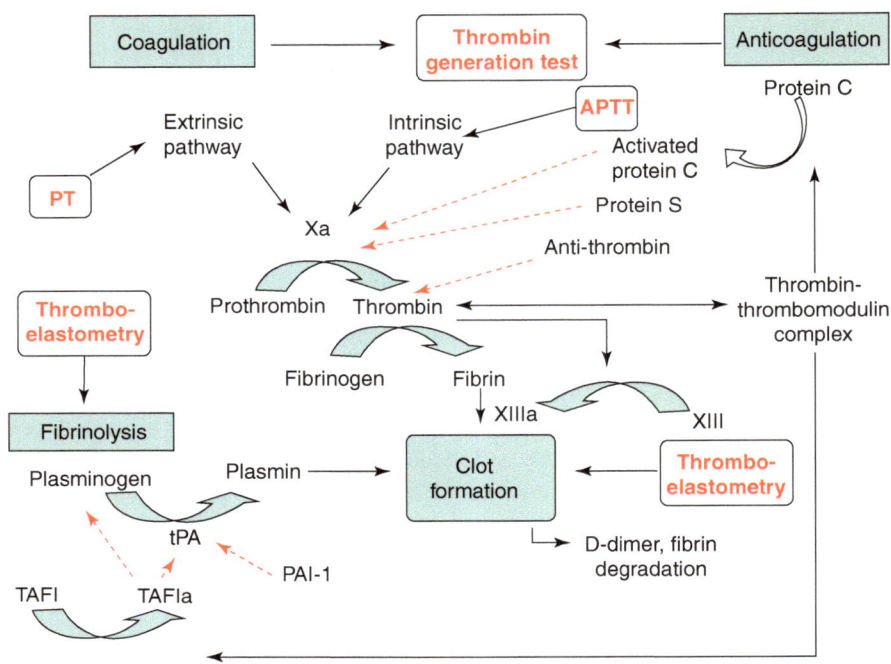

Fig. 12.1 Schematic representation of the coagulation cascade demonstrating the interplay between coagulation, anticoagulation, clot formation and fibrinolysis. *Grey boxes* with *red text* indicate which components of the cascade are measured by that particular test; *dashed red arrows* indicate an inhibitory effect

12.3   The Coagulopathy of Liver Cirrhosis

Cirrhosis is a complex acquired disorder of haemostasis. Under normal circumstances, coagulation is dependent upon an interplay between several opposing pro- and anticoagulant drivers which maintain physiological haemostasis. The end product of coagulation is thrombin generation, which cleaves soluble fibrinogen into fibrin to form a blood clot [15] (Fig. 12.1). Patients with liver cirrhosis have multiple defects in these pathways including deficiencies in both pro- and anticoagulant factors [16], anaemia [17], thrombocytopenia [18], hypo- and dysfibrinogenaemia [19] as well as hyperfibrinolysis [20], resulting in a complex acquired disorder of haemostasis [14]. These derangements, reflected in conventional coagulation indices and bleeding complications, have led to cirrhosis being regarded a prototypical haemorrhagic disorder. However, recent evidence has challenged this interpretation leading to a paradigm shift in understanding, in that there is not hypocoagulation in stable cirrhosis but rather "rebalanced haemostasis" such that clot formation is normal provided platelet counts are $>50 \times 10^9$/L. Moreover in advanced liver disease, there appears to be a tendency to a procoagulant state which has even been implicated in the pathogenesis of fibrosis progression.

12.3.1 Haemorrhagic Phenotype of Liver Cirrhosis

The bleeding diathesis is the phenotype that most clinicians in the ICU will be familiar with. Variceal bleeding is severe and life threatening, often resulting in massive transfusion. There is a long-standing dogma that patients with cirrhosis are "auto-anticoagulated", based not only on an abnormal prothrombin time but also on the frequent occurrence of bleeding. Bleeding can range from trivial to life threatening including cutaneous, gingival or variceal bleeding and also menorrhagia or epistaxis. Factors contributing to bleeding can be considered in terms of defects in pathways of the coagulation cascade and other factors. Cirrhosis is characterised by a reduction in synthesis of all procoagulant factors, the exception being the powerful procoagulant factor VIII, which shows the opposite trend and is also synthesized in extrahepatic sites including the pulmonary vascular endothelium [21]. Platelet levels are important initiators of coagulations since their surface phospholipids provide the platform for assembly of coagulation factors. Whilst platelet numbers and function may be reduced, there is some evidence that platelet hyperactivation may compensate for this [22], perhaps in part due to increased circulating platelet-derived procoagulant microvesicles [23, 24] but also due to elevated levels of the platelet adhesion protein von Willebrand factor and reduced levels of its cleaving protease ADAMTS13 [25]. Finally, anaemia and excessive fibrinolysis may also impair response to bleeding or promote it.

Other factors which promote bleeding include sepsis, endotoxaemia and uraemia [14]. Infection is known to precipitate bleeding and use of antibiotics following variceal haemorrhage has been shown both to reduce severity of bleeding and early rebleeding in randomised trials [26, 27]. Infection has been associated with increased circulating heparinoids in patients with cirrhosis and active bleeding, which may indirectly interfere with coagulation [28]. Uraemia, which may be a result of concomitant renal impairment in patients with cirrhosis, may also contribute to a bleeding tendency due to abnormal platelet-vessel wall interactions and platelet dysfunction [29, 30].

12.3.2 Propensity Towards Thrombosis in Liver Cirrhosis

Thromboses in the portal and mesenteric vasculature are not uncommon in cirrhosis [31] and are thought to be mainly due to sluggish blood flow through the liver due to intrahepatic portal hypertension. However, recent population-based studies have described an increased risk of peripheral venous thrombotic events such as deep vein thrombosis and pulmonary emboli in patients with cirrhosis [32–34], a phenotype which is less recognized by most clinicians. Aside from derangements in the coagulation cascade, other recognised factors may contribute towards the risk of thromboembolism including immobility, hospitalisation and increasing age. Occurrence of an increased risk of these macro-thrombotic complications in cirrhosis is counterintuitive, due to the haemorrhagic complications observed in clinical practice, as well as conventional coagulation indices suggesting hypo-coagulation. This paradox may be better appreciated with an understanding of the tests used to measure deranged coagulation. Conventionally, assessment of coagulation

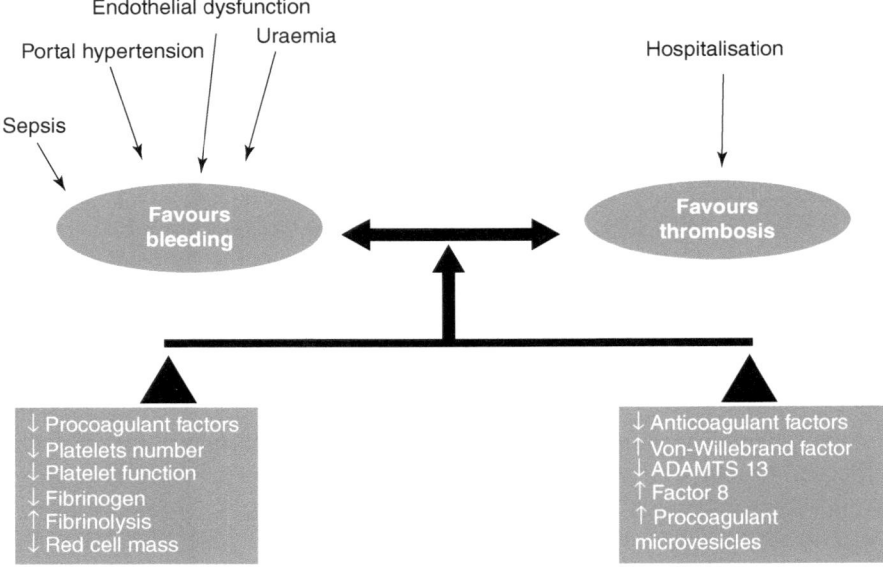

Fig. 12.2 Factors promoting bleeding and thrombosis in liver cirrhosis. The haemostatic balance in liver cirrhosis is precarious and can be easily tipped into a bleeding or thrombotic tendency with an appropriate trigger (Reproduced from *Gut*, Jairath and Burroughs, volume 62 (4), pages 479–82 with permission from BMJ publishing Ltd)

status is based upon evaluation of the prothrombin time (PT), which is only sensitive to thrombin generation with respect to procoagulant factors and is insensitive to the inhibition of thrombin by anticoagulant factors [35]. Therefore, it is not surprising that the PT does not predict the risk of bleeding from varices, nor after invasive procedures, in patients with cirrhosis [36–38], but nonetheless is routinely used to guide transfusion.

More accurate global tests of coagulation include thrombin generation assays and thromboelastography/thromboelastometry, which have shown that plasma from patients with stable (non-bleeding) cirrhosis appears to be normal – hypercoagulable in comparison to healthy controls [16, 39], leading to the concept of "rebalanced haemostasis" [40], albeit a balance which is precarious and may lead to bleeding, thrombosis or even both (Fig. 12.2).

12.4   The Practice of Transfusion of Blood Components for Variceal Bleeding

There are no specific clinical guidelines for the transfusion management of variceal bleeding in cirrhosis. Indeed expert consensus guidelines for the management of variceal bleeding (Baveno guidelines) refrain from making any recommendations on transfusion thresholds given the lack of an evidence base. Two large epidemiological surveys from the UK have characterised actual transfusion practice for AVH.

12.4.1 UK National Audit of the Use of Blood Components in Acute Upper GI Bleeding

In this large nationwide audit, the majority of patients were transfused with RBCs (73 %), and the median haemoglobin (Hb) prior to transfusion was 8.1 g/dL (range 6.9–9.3) with a median of 4 units transfused in total (range 3–6). There was considerable practice variation; for example, in patients with a presenting of Hb >8 g/dL and no evidence of haemodynamic shock, 35 % were transfused with RBCs within 12 h of presentation; conversely 37 % of patients with a presenting Hb > 8 g/dL with evidence of haemodynamic shock were not transfused with RBCs. Fresh frozen plasma (FFP) was transfused in 35 % of patients with a median of 4 units per patient (range 2–6 units); the median INR prior to transfusion of FFP was 1.8 (1.3–2.1), and the median prothrombin time (PT) prior to transfusion was 20 (range 16–22). Seventeen per cent were transfused with FFP in the presence of a normal coagulation screen (INR $\leq$1.5 and/or PT < 3 s prolonged), whereas 41 % with an abnormal coagulation screen (INR > 1.5 and/or PT < 3 s prolonged) were not transfused with FFP. Platelets were transfused to 14 % (76/526) of presentations who were prescribed a median of 2 pools of platelets with a median platelet count prior to transfusion of 43 (IQR 30–62). Of those receiving platelet transfusion, 38 % (29/76) had a platelet count of >50. Overall, 7 % were transfused with cryoprecipitate.

12.4.2 UK National Audit of the Use of Blood Components in Liver Cirrhosis

This national project was undertaken in 2013 to establish patterns of use of blood components in liver cirrhosis. Data was collated on 1,313 consecutive admissions with cirrhosis from 85 hospitals recording all transfusions, whether administered for prophylaxis or treatment of bleeding. In the 192 cases of a variceal bleed, a remarkably similar pattern of transfusion was observed in comparison to the earlier audit in 2007; 92 % received RBCs, and in 54 % of those transfused, the presenting Hb was >7 g/dL. FFP was transfused in 32 % cases, and the pre-transfusion INR was <1.5 in 40 % of cases. Platelets were transfused to 14 % patients, and 46 % of cases had a platelet count of $>50 \times 10^9$. Cryoprecipitate was transfused to 4 % cases. No patients were administered recombinant factor VII, and <5 % received antifibrinolytics.

12.5 Efficacy of Red Blood Cell Transfusion for Gastrointestinal Bleeding

12.5.1 Purpose of RBC Transfusion

During acute bleeding the priority is prompt restoration of circulating volume with intravenous fluids and RBCs to maintain regional and global tissue oxygenation, followed by definitive therapies to control bleeding and to prevent rebleeding (endoscopic, pharmacological and occasionally surgery/radiology). There is limited evidence available on which types of patients benefit from RBCs after AUGIB, at what threshold they should receive them and how much they should receive [41]. Most presentations with AUGIB do not have major bleeding or even features of haemodynamic compromise [42]. Furthermore, 70–80 % cases of AUGIB, especially non-variceal UGIB, will cease spontaneously without the need for endoscopic intervention [43, 44]. Hence, in the majority of cases, RBCs are transfused because the Hb has fallen below a threshold at which the risk of anaemia is perceived to outweigh the risks of transfusion. This threshold is influenced by many factors including the desire to have a "safe" Hb level in the event of rebleeding, to reduce symptoms of anaemia after bleeding has arrested, or by patient-related factors [45]. There is considerable practice variation with respect to RBC transfusion following AUGIB, with rates of transfusion ranging from 23 to 84 % across 208 hospitals in the UK [42].

12.5.2 Guidelines for RBC Transfusion in AUGIB

The evidence base to inform the transfusion recommendations in AUGIB guidelines is sparse and has largely arisen from rodent studies, observational studies and a small number of randomised controlled trials [46]. International consensus guidelines on the management of patients with non-variceal upper GI bleeding advocate a restrictive approach to transfusion using an Hb threshold of ≤ 7 g/dL [47], although this recommendation was based upon trials only conducted in critically ill patient cohorts, where acute bleeding was specifically excluded. Transfusion requirements may be reasonably expected to differ after acute bleeding due to rapid anaemia, haemodynamic compromise and lower Hb levels. Of particular concern in extrapolating this for AUGIB is the high burden of comorbidity, specifically overt and occult cardiovascular and ischaemic heart disease [7]. For patients with cirrhosis and bleeding secondary to variceal bleeding and portal hypertension, guidelines recommend maintaining the Hb around 8 g/dL [48].

12.5.3 Observational Studies on RBC Transfusion in AUGIB

The largest observational study of actual transfusion practice for AUGIB (non-variceal and variceal) to date comes from the UK audit of AUGIB in 2007 which showed practice variation as well as some evidence of inappropriate transfusion practice. An analysis of 4,441 patients who underwent in-patient endoscopy found that after statistical adjustment for markers of disease severity, RBC transfusion in patients with an Hb > 8 g/dL was associated with a twofold increased risk of further bleeding [49]. Similar results were reported in a Canadian study [50]. Whilst these observational studies suggest an association between RBC transfusion and adverse outcome after AUGIB (e.g. further bleeding), they do not prove a causal relationship, since there is a high likelihood of residual confounding in the analyses that arises due to more liberal administration of RBC to sicker patients. However, they provide an important basis to further develop the evidence base for the use of RBCs in AUGIB, by providing data to inform the design of randomised controlled trials (RCTs) of differing transfusion strategies to confirm or refute the findings of these observational studies [51].

12.5.4 Randomised Trial Evidence

A small trial conducted in the UK in 1986 was the first to suggest a causal link between early RBC transfusion after AUGIB and an increased risk of rebleeding, which the authors postulated was the result of transfusion reversing the hypercoagulable response to haemorrhage [52]. A Cochrane review of RCTs identified only three small trials in total comparing differing RBC transfusion strategies in patients with AUGIB from which no firm conclusions could be made [46].

A seminal trial of restrictive versus liberal RBC transfusion for AUGIB was published in 2013 [53]. This was conducted in a single-centre specialised bleeding unit in Spain and randomised over 900 patients into a trial of restrictive (transfusion when Hb <7 g/dL) versus liberal (transfusion when Hb <9 g/dL) RBC transfusion strategies. There were notable exclusion criteria including patients with a history of acute coronary syndrome, peripheral vascular disease, stroke or transient ischaemic attack. There were strict protocols of care within the trial in terms of the use and timing of endoscopy (all patients received endoscopy within 6 h of presentation), pharmacological therapies, administration of single units of RBCs and frequency of haemoglobin concentration measurements [51, 53]. The rates of further bleeding were significantly lower in the restrictive transfusion arm (10 % vs. 16 %), and mortality at 45 days was also lower in the restrictive transfusion arm (5 % vs. 9 %). The treatment effect for mortality was only significant for patients with milder liver cirrhosis and not for patients with peptic ulcer bleeding (which formed almost 50 % of patients in the trial). The rate of overall adverse events was greater in the liberal transfusion arm (48 % vs. 40 %), the key differences being an increase transfusion-associated circulatory overload (TACO) and transfusion reactions in the liberal arm.

This trial has provided a causal relationship between more liberal RBC transfusion after AUGIB and further bleeding and especially produces RCT evidence for the first time to support the age-old dogma of not "overtransfusing" variceal bleeds. However, caution must be exercised in generalising the findings of these results to all patients with AUGIB. Firstly, the stringent processes of care in the trial should be considered when extrapolating the results to each clinician's own institution, especially the ability to provide therapeutic endoscopy within 6 h for all patients no matter what time or day they are admitted, since the availability of such an intervention may in turn influence transfusion thresholds. Secondly, the trial excluded patients with a history of ischaemic heart disease, vascular disease or stroke; given AUGIB is predominantly a disease of older patients, this would exclude almost 40 % of patients presenting in the UK based upon data from the UK audit in 2007 [54]. The optimum transfusion strategy for this group of patients at especially high risk of mortality remains unclear, and therefore a transfusion threshold of 7 g/dL cannot be advocated without further evidence [51]. Recent UK national institute for clinical excellence

(NICE) guidelines for AUGIB acknowledge that further evidence is needed before universally extrapolating restrictive transfusion to all patients with AUGIB.

12.6   Mechanisms of Harm of RBCs for AUGIB

There are many postulated general mechanisms of harm associated with RBC transfusion including transfusion-related immunomodulation and adverse effects associated with ageing RBCs, which also apply to the patient with AUGIB. For patients with cirrhosis and portal hypertensive bleeding, the trial from Barcelona demonstrated in a subgroup of patients that more liberal transfusion was associated with elevated portal pressures, which is a plausible mechanism for both worsening bleeding and promoting rebleeding [53]. This does not explain the mechanism in the vast majority of in the trial who did not have liver cirrhosis. They also postulated that more liberal transfusion may interfere with coagulation to precipitate further bleeding, although this seems implausible with just a mean of two extra RBC units transfused in the liberal transfusion group. The mechanism of increased mortality in the liberal transfusion arm is most likely mediated through further bleeding, since this event is a strong and independent predictor of death [51].

12.7   Platelet Transfusions in GI Bleeding

Thrombocytopenia per se is common in critically ill patients and found to be a risk factor for bleeding and mortality. The prevalence of mild ($<150 \times 10^{-9}$/L) and moderate ($<50 \times 10^{-9}$/L) thrombocytopenia in adult patients on intensive care units is reported at 40 and 8 %, respectively [55]. Most evidence for the use of platelet transfusions comes from the use of prophylactic transfusion in haematological malignancy. Platelet transfusions are infrequently administered to patients with AUGIB; in the UK audit of AUGIB, just 3 % of all presentations to UK hospitals with AUGIB received platelet transfusion. Several consensus guidelines recommend platelet transfusion below a threshold of 50×10^9 in actively bleeding patients, although the evidence to support this is poor. In the UK audit, 61 % of patients who were actively bleeding with a platelet count of $<50 \times 10^9$ did not receive a platelet transfusion, and 42 % of all platelet transfusions were administered to patients with a platelet count of $>50 \times 10^9$ [42]. This variation and uncertainty in practice is likely to reflect the lack of an evidence base to inform the efficacious use of platelet transfusions for the management of AUGIB. There are special considerations for the use of platelets in patients with AUGIB.

12.7.1 Thrombocytopenia in Cirrhosis and Variceal Bleeding

Thrombocytopenia in patients with liver cirrhosis is due to three main reasons: (1) reduced production (as a result of decreased plasma thrombopoetin levels), (2) platelet sequestration (3) and accelerated platelet turnover. In addition to the absolute reduction in platelet count, there is likely to be a degree of thrombocyto-pathy due to abnormalities of the platelet glycoprotein Ib and defective synthesis of thromboxane A2 [56]. Despite both thrombocytopenia and thrombocytopathy, there is some evidence that highly elevated levels of von Willebrand factor in patients with liver cirrhosis contribute to primary haemostasis under experimental flow con-ditions and it is possible that this mechanism may compensate for defects in platelet number and function in cirrhosis [57]. A previous study of critically ill patients with cirrhosis found that platelet transfusion was the only component to significantly improve thromboelastography parameters [58], which provides some rationale for an interventional study. To date, no clinical studies have addressed whether admin-istration of platelet transfusion to the actively bleeding patient with cirrhosis pro-motes haemostasis. Transfusion of any components should be judicious due to the risk of further exacerbating portal pressure.

12.7.2 Managing Antiplatelet Therapy in Non-variceal Bleeding

Over 40 % of patients are taking either an antiplatelet or NSAID agent prior to hos-pitalisation with non-variceal GI bleeding [54]. Given the burden of cardiovascular comorbidity, a proportion of patients who develop non-variceal bleeding are taking aspirin and/or clopidogrel or other antiplatelets. The effect of these drugs lasts for the duration of the platelet life span (i.e. 7–10 days), and the degree of platelet inhi-bition is affected by other factors such as genetic polymorphisms. There is little information in consensus guidelines to inform interventions to manage bleeding in patients taking antiplatelets. In one pilot study in healthy volunteers, transfusion of two autologous platelet components overcame clopidogrel-induced platelet reactiv-ity, but not ADP-induced platelet aggregation. At present there is no evidence to support the use of platelet transfusions to patients taking antiplatelet agents who present with major gastrointestinal bleeding.

12.8   Plasma Transfusion in GI Bleeding

Almost half of fresh frozen plasma (FFP) transfused in the UK is to critically ill patients [59]. A large UK survey showed that 13 % of critically ill adult patients received FFP during an intensive care admission, and half of these were for the treat-ment of bleeding [59]. In theory, FFP may be a useful intervention for reduction of bleeding severity by improving deranged coagulation by replenishing procoagulant and antifibrinolytic factors lost through acute bleeding by providing a source of fibrin-ogen to promote haemostasis. In real-life practice, FFP is frequently transfused to patients with cirrhosis and variceal bleeding as part of initial resuscitation in response to abnormal standard laboratory coagulation indices on the assumption that patients have impaired procoagulant function [42, 53]. In stable cirrhosis, prolongation of the PT is rarely associated with abnormal global assays of coagulation such as thrombin generation [TG] or thromboelastometry [ROTEM] [40, 60], but it is not clear whether a similar discrepancy exists in the setting of acute haemorrhage. Many clinicians prescribe early FFP to correct assumed bleeding tendency, but the risk-benefit balance between haemostatic correction and potential hypervolaemia is uncertain.

Furthermore, aside from liver disease, the clinical efficacy of FFP has not been clearly demonstrated, either for treatment of bleeding or prophylaxis. There is also evidence that standard FFP doses (12–15 mL/kg) are insufficient to significantly increase individual coagulation factor levels. A large volume of FFP transfusion could increase bleeding severity and rebleeding via a direct effect on portal pressure. A better understanding of coagulation during acute haemorrhage would facilitate a more targeted and rational use of FFP.

12.9   Correcting Coagulopathy in Non-variceal Upper GI Bleeding

The term coagulopathy broadly refers to the impairment of blood coagulation in the face of major bleeding or, alternatively, to the laboratory result of a prolonged coagulation time in critically unwell patients. In major haemorrhage following trauma, there has been considerable recent interest in the importance of recognising and treating coagulopathy soon after presentation by earlier use of FFP [61, 62].

Unlike the trauma literature, there are few data for AUGIB on the prevalence of coagulopathy and its impact upon outcome. In the large UK audit, it was observed that after exclusion of patients with liver cirrhosis, 16 % of presentations met criteria for coagulopathy, defined as an INR > 1.5 [63]. Patients with coagulopathy clearly had greater severity of bleeding and, after risk adjustment, had a five times increased risk of mortality compared to those without coagulopathy. It is unclear if coagulopathy is merely a non-specific marker of critical illness or whether haemostatic correction of coagulopathy may improve outcome. Without accurate diagnostic tests to identify specific defects in the clotting pathway, the management of coagulopathy is based on an assumption that reversal of coagulopathy is beneficial. The clinical efficacy of this approach requires further evaluation.

12.10   Antifibrinolytics in AUGIB

Tranexamic acid (TXA) is a derivative of the amino acid lysine which inhibits fibrinolysis by blocking the lysine binding sites on plasminogen molecules. The knowledge that TXA reduces blood loss in surgery and reduces mortality in traumatic bleeding raises the possibility that it might also be effective for GI bleeding. Fibrinolysis could play an important pathological role in AUGIB due to premature breakdown of haemostatic plugs at sites of mucosal injury.

A meta-analysis of seven trials including 1,754 patients demonstrated a 39 % relative reduction in mortality in patients receiving TXA (RR 0.61, 95 % CI 0.42–0.89) compared to placebo, without increasing the risk of thromboembolic events (Forrest plot in Fig. 12.3) [64]. However, the quality of the trials was poor, and only two had adequate allocation concealment. Most of these trials were conducted prior

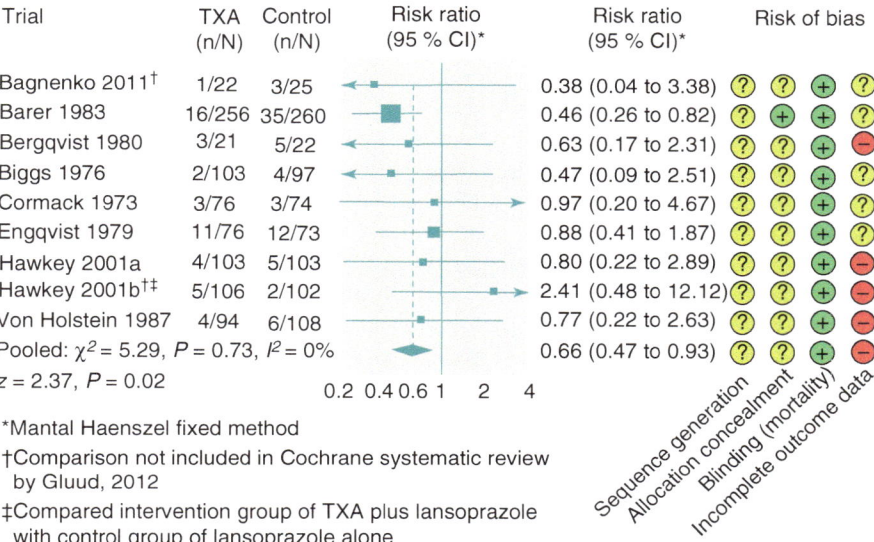

Fig. 12.3 Meta-analysis assessing the effect of tranexamic acid (TXA) on death in acute gastrointestinal bleeding. All trials compare TXA with placebo unless otherwise stated

to the universal use of endoscopic therapy and high-dose proton pump inhibition, which are key features of current management.

Current use of TXA is low. In the UK national audit of upper GI bleeding and the use of blood, only 1 % of patients were given TXA at presentation to the hospital [65]. The effectiveness and safety of TXA for GI bleeding is uncertain, and it is not routinely recommended for treatment in any guideline. A large pragmatic RCT of the effects of TXA on death and transfusion requirement following gastrointestinal haemorrhage is now underway in the UK with results anticipated in 2016.

12.11 Major Haemorrhage Protocols in AUGIB

The advent of major haemorrhage protocols based upon trauma-related massive bleeding has lead to the development of empiric early delivery of FFP and platelets, often in ratio with RBCs of 1:1:1. Massive haemorrhage protocols for trauma should not be extrapolated to patients with AUGIB without careful consideration of whether it is truly major haemorrhage and the potential deleterious consequences. Many patients with AUGIB are elderly with cardiovascular comorbidity and are susceptible to fluid overload. In patients with portal hypertensive bleeding, excessive transfusion volumes risk further elevation of portal pressures and thereby further bleeding.

Take-Home Points for the Practising Clinician Acute upper gastrointestinal bleeding is one of the most common indications for transfusion of all blood components, yet the evidence base to guide safe and effective use of these components is limited. For patients with liver cirrhosis and variceal bleeding, a restrictive approach to RBC transfusion should be followed, with transfusion indicated at thresholds of <7 g/dL, but not higher. However, for other causes of AUGIB, further evidence is needed, and particular caution should be applied in patients with comorbidities such as cardiovascular disease. In patients with liver cirrhosis, conventional coagulation indices such as the prothrombin time do not reflect global haemostasis and these indices should not be used to guide transfusion. There is no evidence that plasma or platelet transfusion should be administered to any patient with gastrointestinal bleeding and the risks of these interventions should be considered before administering them, especially in the patient with portal hypertensive bleeding where injudicious volume administration risks elevating portal pressures and worsening of bleeding and also in those patients with limited cardiac reserve who may not tolerate large volumes of component transfusion. Antifibrinolytics appears to be an effective and safe intervention for AUGIB based upon older trials where they demonstrated a mortality benefit and should be routinely considered until further evidence to the contrary.

References

1. Wells AW, Llewelyn CA, Casbard A, Johnson AJ, Amin M, Ballard S, et al. The EASTR Study: indications for transfusion and estimates of transfusion recipient numbers in hospitals supplied by the National Blood Service. Transfus Med. 2009;19(6):315–28.
2. Tinegate H, Chattree S, Iqbal A, Plews D, Whitehead J, Wallis JP. Ten-year pattern of red blood cell use in the North of England. Transfusion. 2013;53(3):483–9.
3. Crooks C, Card T, West J. Reductions in 28-day mortality following hospital admission for upper gastrointestinal hemorrhage. Gastroenterology. 2011;141:62–70. doi:10.1053/j.gastro.2011.03.048.
4. Lanas A, Garcia-Rodriguez LA, Polo-Tomas M, Ponce M, Alonso-Abreu I, Perez-Aisa MA, et al. Time trends and impact of upper and lower gastrointestinal bleeding and perforation in clinical practice. Am J Gastroenterol. 2009;104(7):1633–41.
5. Jairath V, Barkun AN. Improving outcomes from acute upper gastrointestinal bleeding. Gut. 2012;61(9):1246–9.
6. British Society of Gastroenterology. UK comparative audit of upper gastrointestinal bleeding and the use of blood. http://www.bsg.org.uk/pdf_word_docs/blood_audit_report_07.pdf (2007).
7. Hearnshaw SA, Logan RF, Lowe D, Travis SP, Murphy MF, Palmer KR. Acute upper gastrointestinal bleeding in the UK: patient characteristics, diagnoses and outcomes in the 2007 UK audit. Gut. 2011;60(10):1327–35.
8. Jairath V, Logan R, Hearnshaw S, Travis S, Murphy M, Palmer K. Acute upper gastrointestinal bleeding- why do patients die? Gastroenterology. 2010;138(5;S1):637–8 [Abstract].
9. WHO. Mortality database. Available from: http://www.who.int/healthinfo/morttables/en/index.html (2006).
10. Fleming KM, Aithal GP, Solaymani-Dodaran M, Card TR, West J. Incidence and prevalence of cirrhosis in the United Kingdom, 1992–2001: a general population-based study. J Hepatol. 2008;49(5):732–8.
11. Kovalak M, Lake J, Mattek N, Eisen G, Lieberman D, Zaman A. Endoscopic screening for varices in cirrhotic patients: data from a national endoscopic database. Gastrointest Endosc. 2007;65(1):82–8.

12. North Italian Endoscopic Club for the Study and Treatment of Esophageal Varices. Prediction of the first variceal hemorrhage in patients with cirrhosis of the liver and esophageal varices. A prospective multicenter study. N Engl J Med. 1988;319(15):983–9.
13. Moitinho E, Escorsell A, Bandi JC, Salmeron JM, Garcia-Pagan JC, Rodes J, et al. Prognostic value of early measurements of portal pressure in acute variceal bleeding. Gastroenterology. 1999;117(3):626–31.
14. Jairath V, Burroughs AK. Anticoagulation in patients with liver cirrhosis: complication or therapeutic opportunity? Gut. 2013;62:479–82.
15. Coughlin SR. Thrombin signalling and protease-activated receptors. Nature. 2000;407(6801): 258–64.
16. Tripodi A, Primignani M, Chantarangkul V, Dell'Era A, Clerici M, de Franchis R, et al. An imbalance of pro- vs anti-coagulation factors in plasma from patients with cirrhosis. Gastroenterology. 2009;137(6):2105–11.
17. Thachil J. Anemia–the overlooked factor in bleeding related to liver disease. J Hepatol. 2011;54(3):593–4. author reply 4–5.
18. Pradella P, Bonetto S, Turchetto S, Uxa L, Comar C, Zorat F, et al. Platelet production and destruction in liver cirrhosis. J Hepatol. 2011;54(5):894–900.
19. Francis JL, Armstrong DJ. Acquired dysfibrinogenaemia in liver disease. J Clin Pathol. 1982;35(6):667–72.
20. Ferro D, Celestini A, Violi F. Hyperfibrinolysis in liver disease. Clin Liver Dis. 2009;13(1): 21–31.
21. Jacquemin M, Neyrinck A, Hermanns MI, Lavend'homme R, Rega F, Saint-Remy JM, et al. FVIII production by human lung microvascular endothelial cells. Blood. 2006;108(2): 515–7.
22. Violi F, Basili S, Raparelli V, Chowdary P, Gatt A, Burroughs AK. Patients with liver cirrhosis suffer from primary haemostatic defects? Fact or fiction? J Hepatol. 2011;55(6):1415–27.
23. Sayed D, Amin NF, Galal GM. Monocyte-platelet aggregates and platelet micro-particles in patients with post-hepatitic liver cirrhosis. Thromb Res. 2010;125(5):e228–33.
24. Jairath V, Harrison P, Stanworth S, Collier J, Murphy M, Barnes E. PWE-294 Microparticle dependent procoagulant activity and thrombin generation is increased in patients with cirrhosis induced coagulopathy. Gut. 2012;61 Suppl 2:A417.
25. Mannucci PM, Canciani MT, Forza I, Lussana F, Lattuada A, Rossi E. Changes in health and disease of the metalloprotease that cleaves von Willebrand factor. Blood. 2001;98(9):2730–5.
26. Jun CH, Park CH, Lee WS, Joo YE, Kim HS, Choi SK, et al. Antibiotic prophylaxis using third generation cephalosporins can reduce the risk of early rebleeding in the first acute gastro-esophageal variceal hemorrhage: a prospective randomized study. J Korean Med Sci. 2006; 21(5):883–90.
27. Hou MC, Lin HC, Liu TT, Kuo BI, Lee FY, Chang FY, et al. Antibiotic prophylaxis after endoscopic therapy prevents rebleeding in acute variceal hemorrhage: a randomized trial. Hepatology. 2004;39(3):746–53.
28. Senzolo M, Coppell J, Cholongitas E, Riddell A, Triantos CK, Perry D, et al. The effects of glycosaminoglycans on coagulation: a thromboelastographic study. Blood Coagul Fibrinolysis. 2007;18(3):227–36.
29. Benigni A, Boccardo P, Galbusera M, Monteagudo J, De Marco L, Remuzzi G, et al. Reversible activation defect of the platelet glycoprotein IIb-IIIa complex in patients with uremia. Am J Kidney Dis. 1993;22(5):668–76.
30. Escolar G, Cases A, Bastida E, Garrido M, Lopez J, Revert L, et al. Uremic platelets have a functional defect affecting the interaction of von Willebrand factor with glycoprotein IIb-IIIa. Blood. 1990;76(7):1336–40.
31. Tsochatzis EA, Senzolo M, Germani G, Gatt A, Burroughs AK. Systematic review: portal vein thrombosis in cirrhosis. Aliment Pharmacol Ther. 2010;31(3):366–74.
32. Wu H, Nguyen GC. Liver cirrhosis is associated with venous thromboembolism among hospitalized patients in a nationwide US study. Clin Gastroenterol Hepatol. 2010;8(9):800–5.

33. Sogaard KK, Horvath-Puho E, Gronbaek H, Jepsen P, Vilstrup H, Sorensen HT. Risk of venous thromboembolism in patients with liver disease: a nationwide population-based case-control study. Am J Gastroenterol. 2009;104(1):96–101.

34. Ali M, Ananthakrishnan AN, McGinley EL, Saeian K. Deep vein thrombosis and pulmonary embolism in hospitalized patients with cirrhosis: a nationwide analysis. Dig Dis Sci. 2011;56(7):2152–9.

35. Tripodi A, Mannucci PM. Abnormalities of hemostasis in chronic liver disease: reappraisal of their clinical significance and need for clinical and laboratory research. J Hepatol. 2007;46(4):727–33.

36. Segal JB, Dzik WH. Paucity of studies to support that abnormal coagulation test results predict bleeding in the setting of invasive procedures: an evidence-based review. Transfusion. 2005;45(9):1413–25.

37. Terjung B, Lemnitzer I, Dumoulin FL, Effenberger W, Brackmann HH, Sauerbruch T, et al. Bleeding complications after percutaneous liver biopsy. An analysis of risk factors. Digestion. 2003;67(3):138–45.

38. Boks AL, Brommer EJ, Schalm SW, Van Vliet HH. Hemostasis and fibrinolysis in severe liver failure and their relation to hemorrhage. Hepatology. 1986;6(1):79–86.

39. Gatt A, Riddell A, Calvaruso V, Tuddenham EG, Makris M, Burroughs AK. Enhanced thrombin generation in patients with cirrhosis-induced coagulopathy. J Thromb Haemost. 2010;8(9):1994–2000.

40. Lisman T, Porte RJ. Rebalanced hemostasis in patients with liver disease: evidence and clinical consequences. Blood. 2010;116(6):878–85.

41. Jairath V, Kahan BC, Gray A, Dore CJ, Mora A, Dyer C, et al. Restrictive vs liberal blood transfusion for acute upper gastrointestinal bleeding: rationale and protocol for a cluster randomized feasibility trial. Transfus Med Rev. 2013;27(3):146–53.

42. UK Comparative Audit of Upper Gastrointestinal Bleeding and the Use of Blood. British Society of Gastroenterology. Accessed at www.bsg.org.uk/pdf_word_docs/blood_audit_report_07.pdf (2007).

43. Hearnshaw SA, Logan RF, Lowe D, Travis SP, Murphy MF, Palmer KR. Use of endoscopy for management of acute upper gastrointestinal bleeding in the UK: results of a nationwide audit. Gut. 2010;59(8):1022–9.

44. Pang S, Ching J, Lau J, Sung J, Graham D, Chan F. Comparing the Blatchford and pre-endoscopic Rockall score in predicting the need for endoscopic therapy in patients with upper GI hemorrhage. Gastrointest Endosc. 2010;71:1134–40.

45. Jairath V, Kahan BC, Logan RF, Travis SP, Palmer KR, Murphy MF. Red blood cell transfusion practice in patients presenting with acute upper gastrointestinal bleeding: a survey of 815 UK clinicians. Transfusion. 2011;51(9):1940–8.

46. Jairath V, Hearnshaw S, Brunskill SJ, Doree C, Hopewell S, Hyde C, et al. Red cell transfusion for the management of upper gastrointestinal haemorrhage. Cochrane Database Syst Rev. 2010;9, CD006613.

47. Barkun AN. International consensus recommendations on the management of patients with nonvariceal upper gastrointestinal bleeding. Ann Intern Med. 2010;152:101–13.

48. de Franchis R. Revising consensus in portal hypertension: report of the Baveno V consensus workshop on methodology of diagnosis and therapy in portal hypertension. J Hepatol. 2010;53(4):762–8.

49. Hearnshaw SA, Logan RF, Palmer KR, Card TR, Travis SP, Murphy MF. Outcomes following early red blood cell transfusion in acute upper gastrointestinal bleeding. Aliment Pharmacol Ther. 2010;32(2):215–24.

50. Restellini S, Kherad O, Jairath V, Martel M, Barkun AN. Red blood cell transfusion is associated with increased rebleeding in patients with nonvariceal upper gastrointestinal bleeding. Aliment Pharmacol Ther. 2013;37:316–22.

51. Jairath V. Acute upper gastrointestinal bleeding–time for some new triggers? Transfus Med. 2013;23(3):139–41.

52. Blair SD, Janvrin SB, McCollum CN, Greenhalgh RM. Effect of early blood transfusion on gastrointestinal haemorrhage. Br J Surg. 1986;73(10):783–5.

53. Villanueva C, Colomo A, Bosch A, Concepcion M, Hernandez-Gea V, Aracil C, et al. Transfusion strategies for acute upper gastrointestinal bleeding. N Engl J Med. 2013;368(1):11–21.

54. Hearnshaw SA. Acute upper gastrointestinal bleeding in the UK: patient characteristics, diagnoses and outcomes in the 2007 UK audit. Gut. 2011;10:1327–35. doi:10.1136/gut.2010.228437.

55. Stanworth SJ, Walsh TS, Prescott RJ, Lee RJ, Watson DM, Wyncoll DL. Thrombocytopenia and platelet transfusion in UK critical care: a multicenter observational study. Transfusion. 2013;53(5):1050–8.

56. Afdhal N, McHutchison J, Brown R, Jacobson I, Manns M, Poordad F, et al. Thrombocytopenia associated with chronic liver disease. J Hepatol. 2008;48(6):1000–7.

57. Lisman T, Bongers TN, Adelmeijer J, Janssen HL, de Maat MP, de Groot PG, et al. Elevated levels of von Willebrand Factor in cirrhosis support platelet adhesion despite reduced functional capacity. Hepatology. 2006;44(1):53–61.

58. Clayton DG, Miro AM, Kramer DJ, Rodman N, Wearden S. Quantification of thrombelastographic changes after blood component transfusion in patients with liver disease in the intensive care unit. Anesth Analg. 1995;81(2):272–8.

59. Stanworth SJ. The evidence-based use of FFP and cryoprecipitate for abnormalities of coagulation tests and clinical coagulopathy. Hematology Am Soc Hematol Educ Program. 2007;179–86.

60. Tripodi A, Mannucci PM. The coagulopathy of chronic liver disease. N Engl J Med. 2011;365(2):147–56.

61. MacLeod JB, Lynn M, McKenney MG, Cohn SM, Murtha M. Early coagulopathy predicts mortality in trauma. J Trauma. 2003;55(1):39–44.

62. Brohi K, Singh J, Heron M, Coats T. Acute traumatic coagulopathy. J Trauma. 2003;54(6):1127–30.

63. Jairath V, Kahan BC, Stanworth SJ, Logan RF, Hearnshaw SA, Travis SP, et al. Prevalence, management, and outcomes of patients with coagulopathy after acute nonvariceal upper gastrointestinal bleeding in the United Kingdom. Transfusion. 2013;53(5):1069–76.

64. Manno D, Ker K, Roberts I. How effective is tranexamic acid for acute gastrointestinal bleeding? BMJ. 2014;348:g1421.

65. Hearnshaw SA. Use of endoscopy for management of acute upper gastrointestinal bleeding in the UK: results of a nationwide audit. Gut. 2010;59:1022–9. doi:10.1136/gut.2008.174599.

Platelet Transfusion Trigger in the Intensive Care Unit

13

D. Garry, S. Mckechnie, and S.J. Stanworth

Abstract

Acquired platelet abnormalities may result from a change in platelet number or platelet function. Thrombocytopenia is common in critically unwell patients, and causes are often multifactorial in nature. Up to one quarter of critically ill patients receive a platelet transfusion, usually to prevent rather than to treat bleeding. There are several guidelines to help guide clinicians make platelet transfusion decisions, but little is currently understood about the association between absolute platelet number, in vivo platelet function and overall bleeding risk. This chapter summarises the current and limited evidence for prophylactic platelet transfusion triggers in different clinical scenarios in critically unwell adults, children and neonates. Platelet transfusions are biological agents and not without risk. A main treatment for acquired platelet abnormalities remains management of the underlying disorder.

13.1 Introduction

13.1.1 What Are Platelets and Why Are They Important?

Platelets are circulating anucleate disc-shaped cells that originate from megakaryocytes in the bone marrow. They play a vital role in primary haemostasis (the generation of a platelet plug). A specific glycoprotein receptor (GPIb) on the surface of platelets allows platelets to adhere to endothelial bound von Willebrand factor (vWF).

D. Garry • S. Mckechnie
Department of Anaesthetics and Intensive Care, Oxford University Hospitals NHS Trust, John Radcliffe Hospital, Oxford, UK

S.J. Stanworth (✉)
Department of Hematology, NHS Blood and Transplant/Oxford University Hospitals NHS Trust, John Radcliffe Hospital, Oxford, UK
e-mail: simon.stanworth@nhsbt.nhs.uk

© Springer International Publishing Switzerland 2015
N.P. Juffermans, T.S. Walsh (eds.), *Transfusion in the Intensive Care Unit*,
DOI 10.1007/978-3-319-08735-1_13

Activated platelets change shape and secrete a variety of procoagulant factors (e.g. ADP, calcium, serotonin, fibrinogen, lysosomal enzymes and platelet factor 4) at the site of injury. The interaction of platelets with vWF, released enzymes, ADP and thromboxane A2 (TXA_2) promotes platelet aggregation in which fibrinogen links platelets by the activated GPIIb/IIIa receptors resulting in the formation of a platelet plug. This seals the breach in the endothelium at the site of injury and provides a surface for the procoagulant reactions of secondary haemostasis, in which coagulant factors interact to form a stable fibrin clot.

It is important to recognise that haemostasis in vivo results from the complex interplay of vascular endothelium, platelets, a series of soluble coagulation factors known as the coagulation cascade, anticoagulation mechanisms and the fibrinolytic system. Abnormalities in platelet number (thrombocytopenia or thrombocytosis) and/or platelet function are common in critically ill patients. This may result in either impaired primary haemostasis with increased bleeding risk or (paradoxically) a potential prothrombotic state. Complex patterns of coagulopathy where both bleeding and pro-thrombotic tendencies coexist are well recognised in critical illness, predisposing to increased clinical risk of both bleeding and thrombosis concurrently. This chapter will focus on use of platelet transfusions in critical care. Much of the focus will be on adult intensive care units, as inevitably much of the literature is drawn from clinical studies in adults. Two recent systematic reviews have provided much of the framework for this chapter [1, 2].

- Platelet number
  A platelet count is used to describe the number of circulating platelets. Thrombocytopenia is typically defined as a platelet count below 150×10^9/L, with severe thrombocytopenia defined as a platelet count below 20×10^9/L. Thrombocytosis is defined as a platelet count above 450×10^9/L. Thrombocytosis is commonly seen in ICU patients as a result of inflammation, sepsis and trauma.
- Platelet function
  Functional platelet disorders can be associated with a normal, reduced or even elevated platelet count. A variety of assays are available that provide information on platelet function to varying degrees (Table 13.1). These tests can be considered broadly as global screening tests or specific assays. Results should also be considered alongside platelet counts and size and other tests (e.g. vWF). Many platelet function assays except flow have limitations when platelet counts are less than 100×10^9/L.

13.2 Factors Affecting Platelets in Critical Care Patients

Platelet disorders result from a variety of conditions, both congenital (rare) and acquired (Table 13.2). In critically unwell patients, platelet disorders are usually multifactorial in nature and are frequently accompanied by disorders of other elements of normal haemostasis (such as clotting factors or fibrinogen deficiency).

Table 13.1 Assays that measure platelet function

Test	Method of action	Current use
PFA-100 (closure time)	Mimics a bleeding time by forcing whole blood at high shear through holes in a membrane coated with collagen and either epinephrine or ADP. The time taken for the platelet plug to stop flow is measured	Screening assessment of bleeding risk and quality of platelet concentrates; limitations at low platelet counts. Automated, relatively easy to perform but affected by vWF and haematocrit
Aggregometry	Assesses the ability of various agonists to activate platelets and induce platelet aggregation	Light transmission aggregometry often considered the gold standard but technically challenging, and variability in methodology between laboratories
Flow cytometry	Quantification of membrane glycoproteins	Specialist laboratories
Thromboelastograph (TEG)	Viscoelastic – a sample of blood is placed in a rotating cup; as fibrin forms it applies torque to a pin suspended in the cup; the rotation of the pin is converted to an electrical signal. This produces a graph representing clot formation and lysis	Screening: provides limited information on specific platelet function
		Use in surveillance of cardiac surgery patients, trauma patients
Rotational thromboelastography (ROTEM)	Viscoelastic – similar principle to TEG, but cup is stationary and the pin rotates	As per TEG
Other tests		
Impedance platelet aggregometry (IPA), e.g. multiplate system	Assessing antiplatelet therapy	Difficulties standardisation
Free oscillation rheometry	Uses oscillation to measure clotting time and changes in clot elasticity	Recent technology, under evaluation
Thrombolux	Tests platelet quality	Recent technology, under evaluation

13.3 How Common Is Thrombocytopenia and What Are the Clinical Consequences of Thrombocytopenia?

Platelet abnormalities (often in the absolute number of platelets or in platelet function) may manifest with features of abnormal primary haemostasis such as petechiae, mucosal bleeding or rapid oozing from small cuts, but the exact nature of the relationship between severity of thrombocytopenia and bleeding risk is far from clear and varies considerably between patients. Of potential concern in critically

Table 13.2 Disorders of platelets: some causes

Condition	Mechanism
Inherited	
Mostly rare conditions (giant platelet disorders, Wiskott-Aldrich syndrome etc.) [3]	
Acquired	
Drugs	
Aspirin	Irreversible inhibition of cyclooxygenase (COX)
Dipyridamole	Unclear
$P2Y_{12}$ receptor antagonists, e.g. clopidogrel, ticagrelor	Direct inhibition of ADP receptor or P2Y12 receptor
Glycoprotein IIb/IIIa receptor antagonists, e.g. abciximab, tirofiban	Blockade of the GPIIb/IIIa receptor
Nitrates	Nitric oxide mediated
Calcium channel blockers, e.g. nifedipine	Reduced adhesion and aggregation
Heparin	Reduced adhesion. Reduction in numbers in heparin induced thrombocytopenia
Metabolic (hypothermia, acidaemia)	Reduction in platelet function
Liver disease	Reduction in platelet numbers and function
Uraemia	Reduction in platelet function
Trauma	Reduction in platelet function (as part of the coagulopathy of trauma) and numbers (in major haemorrhage)
Sepsis	Reduction in platelet production and increased platelet consumption
Cardiopulmonary bypass	Reduction in platelet numbers and function
Dysproteinaemia (e.g. multiple myeloma)	Reduction in platelet function
Myeloproliferative disorders	Reduction in platelet function

unwell patients is occult bleeding that is not visible externally, such as into a viscus or an enclosed space (e.g. intracranially).

Thrombocytopenia is common in critically ill adult patients. A recent systematic review showed that it is present in 8–68 % of adult patients on admission to the intensive care unit (ICU) and acquired by 13–44 % of patients during their ICU stay [1]. Thrombocytopenia also complicates critical illness in younger age groups: 20–50 % of critically ill neonates develop thrombocytopenia, including 5–10 % with platelet counts less than $50 \times 10^9/L$ [2].

Thrombocytopenia has been independently linked to death in ICU patients, but this association does not establish causality and therefore cannot be used to help guide platelet transfusion [1].

13.4   What Are Platelet Transfusions?

13.4.1 What Is a Bag of Platelets?

Platelets for transfusion are prepared either by centrifugation of whole blood donations or by aphaeresis. An adult equivalent dose is a pool of four platelet donations in the UK. Platelets can be stored for up to 5 days on an agitator at 22° or longer with a process of bacterial screening. One adult pack of platelets has a volume of 250–350 mL. The usual adult (therapeutic) dose is 1 unit (aphaeresis) or 1 pool (pooled). Each pack costs around 250 euros.

13.4.2 What Is the Effect of Platelet Transfusion on Platelet Count?

The effect of platelet transfusion on platelet count is often assessed by changes in platelet count. In five observational studies in critically ill adults [2, 4–7], platelet transfusion resulted in a median increment of 15×10^9/L. However, results vary considerably across patients [3, 4]. Of note, sustained correction of thrombocytopenia to a count above 100×10^9/L was rarely achieved. The increment in platelet count may be short lived because of the short life span of transfused platelets and coexisting consumptive causes, e.g. hypersplenism. What is less clear is how platelet functions impacts clinical outcomes, such as bleeding risk. No one would disagree with the use of platelet transfusions to treat major bleeding in association with thrombocytopenia. The more common practice of transfusing platelets in non-bleeding patients with thrombocytopenia, however, is more debatable.

13.4.3 Are Platelet Transfusions Common?

Platelet transfusions are commonly used in the ICU; 9–30 % of critically ill patients receive a transfusion, approximately 59–68 % of which are used to prevent, rather than to treat, bleeding [4, 8, 9].

13.5   Risks of Platelet Transfusions

The use of platelets is increasing worldwide. In the UK alone, around 266,000 doses (or aphaeresis equivalent units) were transfused in 2010. Platelets for transfusion are biological components, which are a scarce and costly resource. Nonhaemolytic febrile reactions and mild allergic reactions are common with an estimated incidence of 2 and 4 %, respectively. Anaphylaxis occurs rarely (1:20,000–1:50,000 of transfusions) but accounts for ~40 % of the serious adverse events reported [10].

Table 13.3 Summary of serious morbidity from platelet transfusions (2012 SHOT report [10])

Nature of incident	Number of incidents
Bacterial infection	8
Viral infection (hepatitis B)	1
Transfusion-associated lung injury	1
Anaphylaxis	43
Posttransfusion purpura	2
Total	55

As with all blood components, there is a risk of transfusion-transmitted infection. The rate of viral transmission (HIV, HBV, HCV) appears extremely low. Of more concern is the risk of bacterial infection. Transfusion-transmitted bacterial infection (TTBI) has an estimated incidence of 1:10,000 platelet transfusions. The risk of bacterial contamination is higher than for other blood products because, unlike other blood components, platelets are processed and stored at room temperature. Bacterial screening has been introduced to reduce the risk of TTBI. Transfusion-associated lung injury (TRALI) is a life-threatening complication following platelet transfusion and may be recognised more commonly in the ICU. Platelets are more commonly implicated in TRALI than red blood cells.

The hazards of platelet transfusion are well documented. The 2012 Annual Serious Hazards of Transfusion (SHOT) report featured a total of 2,767 incidents, with platelet transfusions implicated in 55 cases (Table 13.3).

13.6   Current Evidence for Platelet Transfusions

13.6.1 Platelet Transfusions in Adults Who Are Not Critically Ill: Prophylactic Transfusion

In non-bleeding, non-ICU patients, current practice for prophylactic platelet transfusions is derived largely from data in haematology patients with chemotherapy-associated thrombocytopenia. A transfusion trigger of 20×10^9/L was widely used, but other studies comparing 10×10^9/L versus 20×10^9/L as thresholds for platelet transfusion showed no increased bleeding risk when 10×10^9/L was used as the trigger. Indeed, several very recent randomised trials have now tested whether a no-prophylaxis policy can be safely followed in selected low-risk patients with haematological malignancies and severe thrombocytopenia. These findings taken together suggest a limited role for platelet transfusions to reduce bleeding risk, even at counts under 10×10^9/L [11].

The use of prophylactic platelet transfusion is not recommended in patients with heparin-induced thrombocytopenia (HIT) or idiopathic thrombocytopenic purpura (ITP) and is contraindicated in patients with thrombotic thrombocytopenic purpura (TTP).

13.6.2 Platelet Transfusions in Adults Who Are Not Critically Ill: Perioperative and Peri-procedural Transfusion

Although there is a paucity of data to support evidence-based practice, it is widely accepted that patients requiring surgery or interventional procedures should have a higher transfusion trigger. For the majority of procedures (e.g. laparotomy, drain insertion) in stable, non-bleeding patients, the platelet count should be at least 50×10^9. For procedures in critical sites [13] (e.g. brain, eye), the platelet count should be at least 100×10^9.

For neuraxial blockade, published guidance stratifies the risk of bleeding complications (spinal haematoma) in patients with isolated thrombocytopenia and normal platelet function. A platelet count $>75 \times 10^9$ is categorised as normal risk, $50-75 \times 10^9$ increased risk, $20-50 \times 10^9$ high risk and $<20 \times 10^9$ as very high risk. A platelet count of $<50 \times 10^9$ is widely accepted as an absolute contraindication to neuraxial blockade [14].

13.6.3 Platelet Transfusions in Adults Who Are Not Critically Ill: Transfusion Because of Bleeding

There is general consensus that the platelet count should be kept above 50×10^9 in patients who are actively bleeding [15]. In massive haemorrhage, guidelines suggest this trigger is raised to 75×10^9/L [16]. A target level of 100×10^9/L has been recommended in patients with polytrauma or central nervous injury [13]. In major trauma, platelets have increasingly been administered empirically early in the resuscitation as part of a protocolised 1:1:1 red cell to fresh frozen plasma (FFP) to platelet strategy. The evidence for this ratio-driven resuscitation is largely based on observational data in military settings [17]. This data may be influenced by survival bias, and the optimal ratio guiding the administration of platelets in this setting remains contested.

It is clear that most recommendations for the use of platelet transfusion are based on platelet count rather than platelet function. Patients with congenital and/or acquired platelet dysfunction may require platelet transfusion despite a normal platelet count. These patients should have platelet function assessed and are best managed with haematology advice.

13.6.4 Platelet Transfusions in Critically Ill Adults

The following clinical scenario illustrates an example of the type of case seen. Table 13.4 provides a pragmatic summary of recommendations for different platelet count thresholds prior to platelet transfusion.

A 34-year-old has been in the ICU for 6 days with multi-organ failure secondary to biliary sepsis. He is intubated and has an ongoing inotropic requirement. His platelet count has slowly decreased since admission, and today is 17×10^9/L. He has no signs of bleeding. You contemplate whether to administer a prophylactic platelet transfusion.

Table 13.4 Suggested indications for use of platelet transfusions

Patient population	Indication	Transfusion trigger
Adults who are not critically ill	Prophylactic platelet transfusion	10×10^9/L
	Neuraxial blockade	75×10^9/L
	Perioperative transfusion	50×10^9/L
	Perioperative transfusion in critical sites	100×10^9/L
	Bleeding patients	50×10^9/L
Adults who are critically ill	Prophylactic platelet transfusion	$10–20 \times 10^9$/L
	Massive haemorrhage	75×10^9/L
	Polytrauma/CNS injury	100×10^9/L

Although up to 30 % of patients in critical care receive a platelet transfusion, there is little published data to guide best practice on when to transfuse. It appears the majority of transfusions are used to prevent, rather than treat, bleeding complications, but to date, there are no high-quality studies that have looked specifically at platelet transfusions to avoid bleeding in critically ill adults [2]. In the absence of specific data, most recommendations are extrapolated from the recommendations for the general adult population. Suggested platelet transfusion triggers for adults with sepsis are included in the Surviving Sepsis Guidelines [18], but these guidelines reflect consensus opinion with a GRADE IID recommendation. The guidelines suggest a transfusion trigger of 10×10^9/L in the absence of apparent bleeding or 20×10^9/L if a patient has a significant risk of bleeding [18]. The guidelines advocate higher platelet counts ($>50 \times 10^9$/L) for active bleeding, surgery or invasive procedures.

The effect of platelet transfusion on outcome remains unclear. Two studies have shown an association between platelet count recovery (by transfusion or otherwise) and survival [6, 19], but other observational studies have failed to show an association between platelet transfusion and mortality [5–7].

13.6.5 Platelet Transfusions in Critically Ill Neonates and Children

The effect of platelet transfusions on bleeding in neonates has been assessed in nine studies [20–28], but the data are conflicting, and it is difficult to draw clear recommendations on platelet use in this cohort. One study reported a 21 % reduction (95 % confidence interval 8–31) in minor bleeds in the 12 h after platelet transfusion compared with 12 h before transfusion. However, one randomised study reported no difference in mortality or the incidence of intraventricular haemorrhage with a platelet transfusion trigger of 50×10^9/L versus 150×10^9/L. The risk of death among neonates is associated with increased use of platelet transfusions, and data from (unadjusted) observational studies suggest that additional platelet transfusions are associated with a higher incidence of bleeding events. It is likely that the increased risk of death and bleeding events simply reflects the severity of underlying disease, with sicker neonates receiving more platelets.

Given the lack of evidence, it is not currently possible to recommend for or against platelet transfusion in critically ill neonates, at different thresholds of platelet count. Practice in some neonatal units in the UK has seen levels of platelet count thresholds for prophylactic transfusions fall to $20-30 \times 10^9$/L in stable neonates, although many neonatologists might consider higher thresholds in unstable premature neonates in the first week of life. Published guidelines are largely opinion based, which may recommend a transfusion threshold of $25-30 \times 10^9$/L for stable neonates and 50×10^9/L for unstable preterm infants [27, 29, 30]. For term neonates with sepsis, the 2012 Surviving Sepsis Campaign Guidelines advocate the same platelet transfusion triggers as recommended in adults (see above), with a Grade IIC recommendation.

There is little published evidence for the use of platelet transfusions in critically ill children. A prospective cohort study of critically ill children ($n = 138$) reported no difference in mortality between transfused and non-transfused children in adjusted analyses [31]. The 2012 Surviving Sepsis Campaign Guidelines recommended similar platelet transfusion targets in children as for adults in the context of sepsis, with a Grade IIC recommendation.

13.7 Conclusion

Platelet transfusions are commonly used in the ICU. Between 9 and 30 % of critically ill patients receive a transfusion despite a lack of evidence underpinning this intervention. Approximately 59–68 % of platelet transfusions are used to prevent, rather than to treat, bleeding.

Although thrombocytopenia has been independently linked to death in the ICU, the association between low platelet counts and poor clinical outcomes does not establish causality and does not provide adequate evidence to support correction of thrombocytopenia with platelet transfusions.

A platelet count below 20×10^9/L is commonly used to define severe thrombocytopenia in critical illness and often a threshold for administering platelet transfusions in non-bleeding patients. However, the use of a specific platelet count threshold may incorrectly convey that there are stepwise changes in bleeding risk or other outcomes with platelet count alone, which is unlikely to be the case, as many other factors contribute to the maintenance of haemostasis (e.g. fibrinogen). Critically ill patients are heterogeneous with respect to admission diagnoses, co-morbidities, medications and dynamic changes in coagulation parameters. Such factors are, individually or cumulatively, likely to influence both the number and function of platelets and the subsequent overall risk of bleeding. Although stratification of bleeding risk is likely to be more informative than platelet count alone, current data do not yet allow for this, but will be the subject of research over the next few years.

Platelet transfusions are not without risk, and decisions to transfuse depend on several factors in addition to the absolute platelet count. It should be remembered that not all causes of thrombocytopenia are appropriately treated with platelet transfusion (e.g. HIT, TTP, ITP), and the principal treatment for thrombocytopenia in critically ill patients remains treatment of the underlying cause.

References

1. Hui P, Cook DJ, Lim W, Fraser GA, Arnold DM. The frequency and clinical significance of thrombocytopenia complicating critical illness: a systematic review. Chest. 2011;139(2):271–8.
2. Lieberman L, Bercovitz RS, Sholapur NS, Heddle NM, Stanworth SJ, Arnold DM. Platelet transfusions for critically ill patients with thrombocytopenia. Blood. 2014;123(8):1146–51. doi:10.1182/blood-2013-02-435693; quiz 1280. Epub 2013 Dec 12.
3. Roberts I, Stanworth S, Murray NA. Thrombocytopenia in the neonate. Blood Rev. 2008;22(4):173–86.
4. Stanworth SJ, Walsh TS, Prescott RJ, et al. Thrombocytopenia and platelet transfusion in UK critical care: a multicenter observational study. Transfusion. 2013;53(5):1050–8.
5. Arnold DM, Crowther MA, Cook RJ, et al. Utilization of platelet transfusions in the intensive care unit: indications, transfusion triggers, and platelet count responses. Transfusion. 2006;46(8):1286–91. [Erratum appears in Transfusion. 2009;49(9):2012].
6. Stephan F, De Montblanc J, Cheffi A, Bonnet F. Thrombocytopenia in critically ill surgical patients: a case-control study evaluating attributable mortality and transfusion requirements. Crit Care. 1999;3(6):151–8.
7. Stephan F, Hollande J, Richard O, Cheffi A, Maier-Redelsperger M, Flahault A. Thrombocytopenia in a surgical ICU. Chest. 1999;115(5):1363–70.
8. Thomas L, Kaidomar S, Kerob-Bauchet B, et al. Prospective observational study of low thresholds for platelet transfusion in adult dengue patients. Transfusion. 2009;49(7):1400–11.
9. McIntyre L, Tinmouth AT, Fergusson DA. Blood component transfusion in critically ill patients. Curr Opin Crit Care. 2011;19(4):326–33.
10. Bolton-Maggs PHB, editor, Poles D, Watt A, Thomas D, Cohen H, on behalf of the Serious Hazards of Transfusion (SHOT) Steering Group. The 2012 annual SHOT report. 2013.
11. Stanworth SJ, Estcourt LJ, Powter G, Kahan BC, Dyer C, Choo L, Bakhrania L, Llewelyn C, Bielby L, Norfolk D, Wood EM, Murphy MF. The effect of a no-prophylactic versus prophylactic platelet transfusion strategy on bleeding in patients with hematological malignancies and severe thrombocytopenia (TOPPS trial). A randomized controlled, non-inferiority trial. N Engl J Med. 2013;368(19):1771–80.
12. Wandt H, Schaefer-Eckart K, Wendelin K, et al. Therapeutic platelet transfusion versus routine prophylactic transfusion in patients with haematological malignancies: an open-label, multicentre, randomised study. Lancet. 2012;380(9850):1309–16.
13. British Committee for Standards in Haematology, Blood Transfusion Task Force. Guidelines for the use of platelet transfusions. Br J Haematol. 2003;122(1):10–23.
14. Association of Anaesthetists of Great Britain and Ireland, Obstetric Anaesthetists' Association, Regional Anaesthesia UK. Regional anaesthesia and patients with abnormalities of coagulation. Anaesthesia. 2013;68:966–72.
15. Association of Anaesthetists of Great Britain and Ireland. Blood transfusion and the anaesthetist. 2005. http://www.aagbi.org/sites/default/files/bloodtransfusion06.pdf. Accessed 12/03/14.
16. Association of Anaesthetists of Great Britain and Ireland. Blood transfusion and the anaesthetist: management of massive haemorrhage. Anaesthesia. 2010;65:1153–61.
17. Miller TE. New evidence in trauma resuscitation – is 1:1:1 the answer? Perioper Med (Lond). 2013;2(1):13.
18. Dellinger RP, Levy MM, Rhodes A, et al. Surviving Sepsis Campaign: international guidelines for management of severe sepsis and septic shock, 2012. Intensive Care Med. 2013;39(2):165–228.
19. Strauss R, Wehler M, Mehler K, Kreutzer D, Koebnick C, Hahn EG. Thrombocytopenia in patients in the medical intensive care unit: bleeding prevalence, transfusion requirements, and outcome. Crit Care Med. 2002;30(8):1765–71.
20. Andrew M, Vegh P, Caco C, et al. A randomized, controlled trial of platelet transfusions in thrombocytopenic premature infants. J Pediatr. 1993;123(2):285–91.
21. Stanworth SJ, Clarke P, Watts T, et al. Prospective, observational study of outcomes in neonates with severe thrombocytopenia. Pediatrics. 2009;124(5):e826–34.

22. Bonifacio L, Petrova A, Nanjundaswamy S, Mehta R. Thrombocytopenia related neonatal outcome in preterms. Indian J Pediatr. 2007;74(3):269–74.
23. Dohner ML, Wiedmeier SE, Stoddard RA, et al. Very high users of platelet transfusions in the neonatal intensive care unit. Transfusion. 2009;49(5):869–72.
24. Garcia MG, Duenas E, Sola MC, Hutson AD, Theriaque D, Christensen RD. Epidemiologic and outcome studies of patients who received platelet transfusions in the neonatal intensive care unit. J Perinatol. 2001;21(7):415–20.
25. Gerday E, Baer VL, Lambert DK, et al. Testing platelet mass versus platelet count to guide platelet transfusions in the neonatal intensive care unit. Transfusion. 2009;49(10):2034–9.
26. Kahn DJ, Richardson DK, Billett HH. Inter-NICU variation in rates and management of thrombocytopenia among very low birth-weight infants. J Perinatol. 2003;23(4):312–6.
27. Murray NA, Howarth LJ, McCloy MP, Letsky EA, Roberts IAG. Platelet transfusion in the management of severe thrombocytopenia in neonatal intensive care unit patients. Transfus Med. 2002;12(1):35–41.
28. Muthukumar P, Venkatesh V, Curley A, et al. Severe thrombocytopenia and patterns of bleeding in neonates: results from a prospective observational study and implications for use of platelet transfusions. Transfus Med. 2012;22(5):338–43.
29. Gibson BE, Todd A, Roberts I, et al. Transfusion guidelines for neonates and older children. Br J Haematol. 2004;124(4):433–53.
30. Poterjoy BS, Josephson CD. Platelets, frozen plasma, and cryoprecipitate: what is the clinical evidence for their use in the neonatal intensive care unit? Semin Perinatol. 2009;33(1):66–74.
31. Agrawal S, Sachdev A, Gupta D, Chugh K. Platelet counts and outcome in the pediatric intensive care unit. Indian J Crit Care Med. 2008;12(3):102–8.

David Hall and Timothy S. Walsh

Abstract

Coagulopathies are common in the critically ill but are often mild and short lived. Detailed assessment of haemostasis is normal in many of these cases and there is no evidence and little clinical rationale, for transfusing FFP in the absence of bleeding, even when invasive procedures are planned. The risk of procedure-related bleeding is very low, and evidence suggests that prophylactic plasma does not modify risk for most cases. Pre-procedural FFP should be reserved for patients with significantly prolonged INR (>2.5–3.0) undergoing higher-risk procedures. Currently recommended doses of FFP (10–15 mL/kg) do not generate important improvements in INR or APTT, especially when the INR is <2.5. For patients with more significant abnormalities (e.g. INR >3) or where physiological correction is intended because of high-risk procedures (e.g. CNS procedures), a larger dose of FFP (20–30 mL/kg) is required. The significant volume associated with larger doses requires careful consideration of the rate of administration, the patient's intravascular status and the potential risk of transfusion-associated circulatory overload.

14.1   FFP Use in Critical Illness

It is common for patients in the intensive care unit (ICU) to develop disorders of coagulation in association with their critical illness. Up to 30 % of adult patients admitted to ICUs have an INR (international normalised ratio) greater than 1.5 at some point during their admission [1]. This coagulopathy of critical illness is

D. Hall • T.S. Walsh (✉)

Department of Anaesthetics, Critical Care and Pain Medicine, Queens Medical Research Institute, University of Edinburgh, Little France Crescent, Edinburgh EH16 4TJ, UK
e-mail: twalsh@staffmail.ed.ac.uk

© Springer International Publishing Switzerland 2015
N.P. Juffermans, T.S. Walsh (eds.), *Transfusion in the Intensive Care Unit*,
DOI 10.1007/978-3-319-08735-1_14

associated with both acute and chronic liver and kidney disease, sepsis, recent blood transfusion and a higher APACHE II score. Disordered coagulation not only increases the risk of bleeding but also leads to microvascular thrombosis, with resulting end-organ hypoperfusion and dysfunction. Fresh frozen plasma (FFP) is commonly administered to coagulopathic, critically ill patients (between 12.7 and 29.9 %) either as part of the treatment of bleeding or prophylactically to prevent bleeding. This chapter focusses on the use of FFP in the ICU setting, specifically in the absence of major bleeding. The management of major bleeding is dealt with elsewhere.

14.1.1 What Is FFP?

Plasma is the noncellular component of blood and may be prepared by either centrifugation of donated whole blood or by plasmapheresis with leucodepletion. FFP can be produced from single donations or pooled donations. Reduction of infection risk, especially for variant CJD (vCJD) and enveloped viruses (e.g. HIV, HBV, HCV) can be achieved by pathogen-reduction techniques; the two commonest approaches are methylene blue treatment or solvent-detergent treatments. The use of these varies between countries and is driven in part by production policies and the risk of vCJD. An important consideration is that pathogen reduction reduces con-centrations of procoagulant factors, especially fibrinogen and factor VIII (by approximately 30 %) compared to untreated plasma, which decreases efficacy per unit volume.

When frozen within 8 h to −30 °C, plasma is referred to as fresh frozen plasma (FFP). If frozen later (up to 24 h after preparation), it is known as frozen plasma (F24). Both FFP and F24 contain concentrations of clotting factors that are largely equivalent to those found in vivo (with the exception of pathogen-inactivated FFP as noted above), although the concentration of factors V and VIII is lower in F24 due to their instability prior to freezing. The concentration of all plasma proteins is diluted by the sodium citrate solution used as part of the preparation of FFP/F24. Typical factor concentrations in FFP are given in Fig. 14.1. Besides clotting factors,

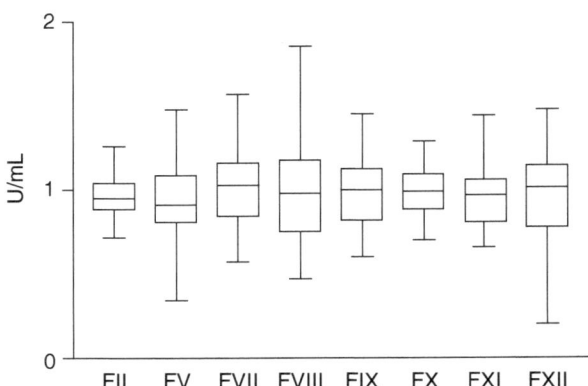

Fig. 14.1 Factor concentrations in white-cell-reduced FFP (Taken from Stanworth et al. [2])

FFP also contains other plasma proteins including acute-phase proteins, von Willebrand factor, donor immunoglobulins and albumin. Donor leukocytes are also present, even following leucodepletion, but at low concentration (typically 1×10^6 leucocytes per component). A typical unit of plasma has a volume of 180–300 mL and may be stored for up to 36 months in most countries. After thawing, the level of factor VIII in plasma falls rapidly, together with factor V levels, but levels of fibrinogen and other haemostatic components are maintained. Guidelines permit the use of plasma that has been thawed for up to 24 h after thawing, but best practice is to order FFP only when required and transfuse it immediately following receipt at the bedside to maximise efficacy. FFP that is not for immediate transfusion following thawing should be stored at 4 °C until transfusion.

14.1.2 Indications for FFP Use in Critical Illness

The use of FFP in critical illness has increased in recent years, although the evidence base supporting its clinical effectiveness is surprisingly lacking. Recommendations in national guidelines [3] are largely based on expert opinion rather than conclusions from well-conducted, randomised trials. Accepted potential indications in critically ill patients include the following:

1. Replacement of multiple coagulation factor deficiencies associated with severe bleeding, disseminated intravascular coagulation and acute traumatic coagulopathy. The treatment of major haemorrhage, in which FFP is administered as part of a protocolised response to massive blood loss, is dealt with in a separate chapter.
2. Correction of coagulopathy in non-bleeding patients.
3. Prophylaxis prior to invasive procedural instrumentation (e.g. central line insertion) in coagulopathic patients.
4. Specific indications, e.g. plasma exchange in thrombotic thrombocytopenic purpura and Guillain-Barre syndrome, treatment of C1-esterase inhibitor deficiency.

   The use of FFP for prophylactic correction of coagulopathy prior to procedures is discussed in more detail below.

14.1.3 Situations in Which FFP Transfusion Is Inappropriate

1. *Reversal of warfarin anticoagulation.* In the absence of bleeding, excessive anticoagulation as a result of warfarin administration should be reversed with intravenous or oral vitamin K. In the presence of bleeding and a prolonged INR in a patient taking warfarin, prothrombin complex concentrate is recommended rather than FFP, which is only partially effective in reversing over-warfarinisation.
2. *Correction of single-factor deficiencies.* In this situation, single-factor concentrate is available and should be used.

3. *Volume expansion.* There is no evidence to support the routine use of FFP as a colloid solution, and the risk/benefit balance and cost-effectiveness have never been explored in adequately powered randomised controlled trials.

In addition, FFP is absolutely contraindicated in congenital IgA deficiency in the presence of anti-IgA antibodies and relatively contraindicated in pulmonary oedema.

14.1.4 FFP Use During Critical Illness

Observational studies indicate that approximately 30 % of critically ill patients experience an episode of INR prolongation, although in the majority of cases (70–75 %) the worst INR is less than 2.5, and abnormalities are limited to a single abnormal test result [1, 7]. Despite this, 30 % of episodes of prolonged INR were associated with FFP prescription (10–15 % of all ICU admissions). Typically, 50 % of FFP prescriptions are given to non-bleeding patients, of which half are administered prior to a procedure and half to treat coagulopathy despite no procedure. Observational studies show wide variation in practice, and in response to surveys, clinicians indicate wide variation in beliefs about use of FFP in the absence of bleeding. Clinicians appear more likely to administer pre-procedural FFP when patients have liver disease and other coagulation abnormalities (low platelets; prolonged APTT) or are receiving concurrent red cell transfusions [8, 9].

Observational studies indicate wide variation in FFP dose between clinicians. Concurrent bleeding is associated with higher clinical doses. However, many clinicians prescribe smaller doses than recommended in current guidelines (see below).

14.2   Tests to Assess the Risk of Bleeding

The most commonly used laboratory assay of coagulation factor activity is the prothrombin time (PT). This provides a measure of the extrinsic pathway of coagulation and represents the time taken for plasma to clot after the addition of tissue factor (Factor III). The PT may be standardised to calculate a prothrombin ratio or international normalised ratio (INR). PT ratio is calculated as PT ratio = PT/MNPT and INR as INR = $(PT/MNPT)^{ISI}$, in which MNPT and ISI are the local, laboratory-specific mean normal PT and international specificity index, respectively. Calculating INR therefore provides an adjustment for different thromboplastin sensitivities between different laboratories.

Despite a lack of robust evidence, an INR of greater than 1.5 is frequently recommended as the threshold for considering FFP transfusion and is present in most guidelines. This cut-off is associated with impending haemostatic failure and represents a fall in the activity of some coagulation factors to less than 50 % of normal. As can be seen from Fig. 14.2, there is significant functional reserve in normal coagulation factor levels, and even at an INR of 1.5, there may be normal haemostasis as

Fig. 14.2 Relationship between coagulation factor concentration and PR/INR (Taken from Yazer et al. [4])

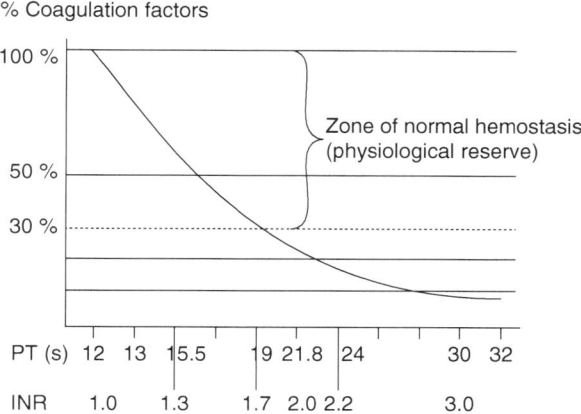

measured by concentrations of individual factor levels. Significant bleeding risk is thought to be increased only when factor levels are less than 30 % of normal ranges. However, this number relates to a single-factor deficiency and may not hold for conditions characterised by multiple factor deficiencies.

There are several well-recognised disadvantages to making FFP transfusion decisions based on PT or INR. In vitro laboratory coagulation tests poorly reflect the complex in vivo haemostatic milieu [5], and there are relatively few studies that support a link between a prolonged PT/INR and bleeding [6]. The long lead time between drawing a sample from a patient to receiving the INR test result (typically in the order of 45 min in many hospitals) means that in a rapidly changing clinical situation, the INR result no longer reflects the patient's current haemostatic status by the time the result is available. Transfusion of FFP in coagulopathic patients, especially those without bleeding, typically results in no change or only a modest improvement in INR when currently recommended doses of 10–15 mL/kg are administered. For example, an 11 mL/kg transfusion of FFP in adults reduced median INR by only 0.2 [7]. Observational data indicates that correction of INR (or equivalent) rarely occurs when the INR is in the 1.5–2.5 range; larger corrections are typically observed at progressively greater derangements. However, correction is typically short lived and limited to less than 24 h.

As the use of point of care, whole-blood viscoelastic tests of coagulation (e.g. ROTEM®/TEG®) increases, it may be possible to recommend thresholds for FFP transfusion based on the results of these technologies. By providing a faster turn-around and allowing the quantification of the interaction between coagulation factors, platelets and red cells in whole blood (rather than utilising plasma only, as with PT and APTT), these tests have several attractive advantages. It is now common-place to make blood product transfusion decisions in the resuscitation of major trauma based on viscoelastic ROTEM®/TEG® results. There is as yet limited evidence for translating this to non-bleeding patients in intensive care units.

14.3   Utility of FFP During Coagulopathy and in Relation to Invasive Procedures

Invasive procedures such as central venous catheterisation or percutaneous tracheostomies are common in patients admitted to intensive care units. These are potentially associated with bleeding, which could have significant morbidity. Such patients, although not necessarily bleeding, frequently have deranged tests of coagulation. The potential consequences of bleeding depend significantly on the site and nature of the procedure but are generally considered higher in relation to the central nervous system (closed spaces), tracheostomy and major organ biopsy. Other factors such as operator experience and expertise are also relevant. FFP is frequently prescribed with the intention of reducing the likelihood and severity of peri-procedural bleeding.

Observational studies indicate significant variation in use of FFP in relation to procedures between clinicians, ICUs and countries. One case-controlled study found that patients with chronic liver disease, thrombocytopenia or receiving concurrent red cell concentration transfusion were all more likely to be prescribed FFP in relation to central venous cannulation [8, 9].

14.3.1 Dose Recommendations

Endogenous factor concentrations of 25–30 % are typically sufficient for haemostasis. Given a typical plasma volume of 40 mL/kg, dose recommendations are therefore 10–15 mL/kg FFP, which equates to 2–4 units (600–1,200 mL) for most adults [10]. Despite these guidelines, larger doses of 20–30 mL/kg are required to reliably increase individual factor levels; these doses represent significant FFP volumes which may increase the risk of hypervolaemia and TACO in non-bleeding patients.

14.3.2 Evidence-Based FFP Transfusion

Despite being common practice, the evidence base supporting FFP transfusion in non-bleeding patients prior to an invasive procedure or as prophylaxis is weak, with few high-quality studies supporting this practice. A Cochrane systematic review recently found no trials meeting predefined quality criteria that compare a liberal with a restrictive transfusion strategy for FFP use in critically ill patients [11]. Current recommendations are therefore largely based on consensus and expert opinion.

Excluding massive trauma, there is no high-quality evidence that plasma transfusion confers a benefit on mortality [12]. In observational studies, the receipt of FFP is associated with higher mortality, even after adjustment for potential confounders, but these cohort studies are subject to "bias by indication". There is little evidence that abnormal coagulation tests predict peri-procedural bleeding in critically ill patients, especially for vascular catheterisation [6]. The available evidence for this predominantly relates to observational and other low-quality studies. These suggest

Table 14.1 Factors that may increase justification for using pre-procedural FFP in critically ill patients

Factor	Clinical rationale
INR >2.5–3.0	Individual factor levels are frequently >30 % normal values, consistent with normal haemostasis, when INR is <2.5
Complex coagulopathy	Concurrent thrombocytopenia or DIC may increase bleeding risk
High-risk procedure	Central nervous system procedure
	Biopsy of organ or site with high risk of bleeding or in which consequences of bleeding may be life threatening (e.g. lung, liver)
	Technically difficult procedure anticipated
Evidence of significantly abnormal clot formation	Dynamic tests of clot formation using ROTEM®/TEG® may be useful for discriminating patients at higher risk of bleeding (but evidence to support this is circumstantial)
Concurrent bleeding in a patient with abnormal INR	Loss of factor levels

that central venous cannulation, one of the most common procedures undertaken on critically ill patients, is not associated with significant bleeding in the context of deranged coagulation [13–15]. The increasing use of ultrasound may also modify the risk between coagulopathy and procedural bleeding, but this has not been demonstrated and factors such as operator skill and experience are also important. Similarly, the rate of bleeding in patients undergoing bronchoscopy, percutaneous tracheostomy and thoracocentesis is similar in patients with both normal and deranged coagulation tests. However, the quality of available evidence is low, and the consequences of bleeding and risk-to-benefit ratio within individual patients is a major consideration. Minor bleeding in a noncompressible and/or critical site (e.g. post intracranial bolt insertion) is more serious than that from a compressible bleed following internal jugular vein catheterisation.

Together these data do not support routine use of FFP for patients with prolonged INR or APTT prior to invasive procedures in the ICU. This is particularly the case for central venous catheterisation. The factors that may increase clinical justification for pre-procedural FFP are listed in Table 14.1.

Studies that measured individual factor levels following different doses of FFP in critically ill patients, together with the absence of correction of INR following most FFP transfusions, support the use of higher FFP doses (20–30 mL/kg) when pre-procedural correction is considered necessary.

14.4   Risks Associated with FFP Transfusion

The administration of FFP to critically ill patients is not without risk, and transfusion-associated circulatory overload (TACO), transfusion-related acute lung injury (TRALI) and allergic reactions are all associated with FFP. TACO and TRALI are considered elsewhere. Both anaphylactic (e.g. secondary to ABO incompatibility) and anaphylactoid reactions (secondary to residual donor plasma protein, platelets or leucocytes) are associated with FFP transfusion. More mild allergic reactions to FFP may occur in as many as 3 % of all FFP transfusions. Infectious diseases can also be transmitted by FFP, although this is rare because of screening and pathogen inactivation.

14.5   Summary

Prolongation of the INR and APTT is common in the critically ill. In most patients, the derangement is mild and short lived; haemostasis is normal in many of these cases. There is no evidence and little clinical rationale, for transfusing FFP to a non-bleeding patient in whom no procedure is planned. For most procedures, the risk of clinically important bleeding in patients with prolonged INR or APTT is extremely low, and in the absence of high-quality evidence, the risk to benefit balance does not support administration of FFP. Pre-procedural FFP should be reserved for patients with significantly prolonged INR (>2.5–3.0) undergoing higher-risk procedures, including those where the risk from bleeding is high.

Currently recommended doses of FFP (10–15 mL/kg) do not generate important improvements in INR or APTT, especially when the INR is <2.5. This may be in part because these patients do not have haemostatic abnormalities. For patients with more significant abnormalities (e.g. INR >3) or where physiological correction is intended because of high-risk procedures (e.g. CNS procedures), a larger dose of FFP (20–30 mL/kg) is required. The significant volume associated with larger doses requires careful consideration of the rate of administration, the patient's intravascular status and the potential risk of TACO.

References

1. Walsh TS, Stanworth SJ, Prescott RJ, Lee RJ, Watson DM, Wyncoll D. Prevalence, management, and outcomes of critically ill patients with prothrombin time prolongation in United Kingdom intensive care units. Crit Care Med. 2010;38(10):1939–46.
2. Stanworth SJ. The evidence-based use of FFP and cryoprecipitate for abnormalities of coagulation tests and clinical coagulopathy. Hematology. 2007;1:179–86.
3. Iorio A, Basileo M, Marchesini E, Materazzi M, Marchesi M, Esposito A, et al. The good use of plasma. A critical analysis of five international guidelines. Blood Transfus. 2008;6(1):18–24.
4. Yazer MH. A primer on evidence-based plasma therapy. ISBT Sci Ser. 2012;7(1):220–5.
5. Holland L, Sarode R. Should plasma be transfused prophylactically before invasive procedures? Curr Opin Hematol. 2006;13(6):447–51.
6. Segal JB, Dzik WH, Transfusion Medicine/Hemostasis Clinical Trials Network. Paucity of studies to support that abnormal coagulation test results predict bleeding in the setting of invasive procedures: an evidence-based review. Transfusion. 2005;45(9):1413–25.
7. Stanworth SJ, Walsh TS, Prescott RJ, Lee RJ, Watson DM, Wyncoll D, et al. A national study of plasma use in critical care: clinical indications, dose and effect on prothrombin time. Crit Care. 2011;15(2):R108.
8. Hall DP, Lone NI, Watson DM, Stanworth SJ, Walsh TS, Intensive Care Study of Coagulopathy (ISOC) Investigators. Factors associated with prophylactic plasma transfusion before vascular

catheterization in non-bleeding critically ill adults with prolonged prothrombin time: a case-control study. Br J Anaesth. 2012;109(6):919–27.

9. Watson DM, Stanworth SJ, Wyncoll D, McAuley DF, Perkins GD, Young D, et al. A national clinical scenario-based survey of clinicians' attitudes towards fresh frozen plasma transfusion for critically ill patients. Transfus Med. 2011;21(2):124–9.

10. O'Shaughnessy DF, Atterbury C, Bolton Maggs P, Murphy M, Thomas D, Yates S, et al. Guidelines for the use of fresh-frozen plasma, cryoprecipitate and cryosupernatant. Br J Haematol. 2004;126(1):11–28.

11. Karam O, Tucci M, Combescure C, Lacroix J, Rimensberger PC. Plasma transfusion strategies for critically ill patients. Cochrane Injuries Group. 2013. doi:10.1002/14651858.CD010654.

12. Murad MH, Stubbs JR, Gandhi MJ, Wang AT, Paul A, Erwin PJ, et al. The effect of plasma transfusion on morbidity and mortality: a systematic review and meta-analysis. Transfusion. 2010;50(6):1370–83.

13. Fisher NC, Mutimer DJ. Central venous cannulation in patients with liver disease and coagulopathy–a prospective audit. Intensive Care Med. 1999;25(5):481–5.

14. Foster PF, Moore LR, Sankary HN, Hart ME, Ashmann MK, Williams JW. Central venous catheterization in patients with coagulopathy. Arch Surg Chic Ill 1960. 1992;127(3):273–5.

15. Doerfler ME, Kaufman B, Goldenberg AS. Central venous catheter placement in patients with disorders of hemostasis. Chest. 1996;110(1):185–8.

Transfusion-Related Acute Lung Injury

15

Alexander P.J. Vlaar and Nicole P. Juffermans

Abstract

Transfusion-related acute lung injury (TRALI) is the leading cause of transfusion-related mortality among critically ill patients. In the absence of biomarkers, the diagnosis is based on clinical parameters. TRALI is defined as onset of acute lung injury (PaO_2/FiO_2 <300, bilateral infiltrates on the chest X-ray) occurring within 6 h of any blood transfusion. Furthermore, hydrostatic pulmonary edema should be ruled out. The incidence of TRALI is high among critically ill patients, which may be due to a "two-hit" pathogenesis of TRALI. The "first hit" is the underlying condition of the patient resulting in priming of the pulmonary neutrophils. The "second hit" is the transfusion of a blood product resulting in activation of the neutrophils and onset of pulmonary edema. Patients with sepsis, hematologic malignancy, cardiac surgery, mechanical ventilation, and massive transfusion are particularly at risk for the onset of TRALI. The mortality of TRALI is up to 50 % in the critically ill patient population. Currently, no specific therapy exists for this life-threatening syndrome. Focus is on prevention and supportive care. Prevention can be achieved by adapting a restrictive and patient-customized transfusion policy, balancing the benefits and risks of transfusion prior to administering a blood product. Supportive care consists out of mechanical ventilation using low tidal ventilation and adapting a restrictive fluid policy.

A.P.J. Vlaar, MD, PhD (✉) • N.P. Juffermans, MD, PhD
Department of Intensive Care Medicine, Laboratory of Experimental Intensive Care and Anesthesiology (L.E.I.C.A.), Academic Medical Center,
Room C3-331, Meibergdreef 9, Amsterdam 1105 AZ, The Netherlands
e-mail: a.p.vlaar@amc.uva.nl

© Springer International Publishing Switzerland 2015
N.P. Juffermans, T.S. Walsh (eds.), *Transfusion in the Intensive Care Unit*,
DOI 10.1007/978-3-319-08735-1_15

15.1 Transfusion-Related Acute Lung Injury: Definition and Pathogenesis

15.1.1 Definition

In the absence of a specific diagnostic test, transfusion-related acute lung injury (TRALI) is defined using a clinical consensus definition (Table 15.1) [1, 2]. In short, TRALI is defined as the onset of acute hypoxia occurring within 6 h after administering any blood transfusion, which cannot be completely explained by the presence of hydrostatic edema. A risk factor for acute lung injury (ALI) should be absent prior to onset of TRALI.

Although this definition appears straightforward, a complicating factor is that the characteristics of TRALI are indistinguishable from ALI due to other causes, such as sepsis, major surgery, or lung contusion. Using this definition would rule out the possibility of diagnosing TRALI in critically ill patients with an underlying ALI risk factor who have also received a transfusion. To identify such cases, the term "possible TRALI" was developed (Table 15.1), which allows for the presence of another risk factor for ALI.

15.1.2 Pathogenesis

TRALI is suggested to be a "two-hit" event [3]. The "first hit" is the underlying condition of the patient resulting in priming of the pulmonary neutrophils. The "second hit" is the transfusion of a blood product. With regard to the causative factors in the blood product, TRALI can be divided in antibody-mediated TRALI and non-antibody-mediated TRALI. Antibody-mediated TRALI is caused by the passive infusion of human leukocyte or human neutrophil antibodies (HLA or HNA) originating from the donor and directed against the antigens of the recipient. Non-antibody-mediated TRALI is caused by the transfusion of stored cellular blood products (red blood cells and platelet concentrates). During storage, proinflammatory mediators accumulate in the blood product. Also, erythrocytes and platelets undergo morphological changes

Table 15.1 Definition of transfusion-related acute lung injury

TRALI
Acute onset within 6 h after a blood transfusion
PaO_2/FiO_2 <300 mmHg
Bilateral infiltrative changes on the chest X-ray
No sign of hydrostatic pulmonary edema (PAOP <18 mmHg or CVP <15 mmHg)
No other risk factor for ALI present
Possible TRALI
Other risk factors for ALI present

PAOP pulmonary arterial occlusion pressure, *CVP* central venous pressure, *ALI* acute lung injury during aging. Both factors have been associated with the onset of TRALI in experimental and observational studies [4–8]. Although the "two-hit" model covers most of the TRALI cases, not all antibody-positive units result in TRALI, even in the presence of the corresponding antigen [9]. Furthermore, antibody-containing blood products were able to induce TRALI in healthy volunteers, i.e., in the absence of a "first hit" [10, 11]. For this reason, a threshold model has been proposed for antibody-mediated TRALI. The threshold model expands on the "two-hit" model by explaining susceptibility of the recipient to develop TRALI [12]. In relatively healthy patients (with a weak "first hit"), a strong antibody incompatibility or high volume of antibodies is needed to overcome the threshold. Conversely, in severely ill patients (with a strong "first hit"), already a weak antibody incompatibility or just a low volume of antibodies is able to overcome the threshold. Both models provide an explanation for the high incidence of TRALI among critically ill patients and have been confirmed by preclinical and clinical studies [13–19].

15.2 Incidence of Transfusion-Related Acute Lung Injury

The incidence of TRALI is high among critically ill patients. The incidence is significantly higher compared to general ward patient populations [20]. An explanation for this difference may be that a "first hit" is often present in critically patients. Furthermore, critically ill patients are often exposed to blood transfusion [21]. The incidence of TRALI in the critically ill has been studied in a few large prospective trials. The estimated incidence of TRALI was around 2% in a cohort of transfused cardiac surgery patients admitted to the ICU [18]. The incidence of TRALI in the general ICU patient population is estimated between 5 and 8 % of transfused patients [13, 17]. Patients admitted to the ICU because of a gastrointestinal bleeding have the highest reported incidence of TRALI, with up to 15 % in transfused patients [22]. In comparison, studies performed in patient populations on the general ward and national hemovigilance reports show incidences of TRALI varying between 0.001 and 0.01 % per product transfused, while ICU studies report up to 1 % per product transfused [15, 23].

15.3 Risk Factors for Transfusion-Related Acute Lung Injury

15.3.1 Patient-Related Risk Factors

It is conceivable that risk factors for ALI are also risk factors for TRALI, given that the "two-hit" model of TRALI holds that priming of lung neutrophils at the time of transfusion can occur by a proinflammatory response of any origin (Table 15.2) [12]. Risk factors associated with both TRALI and ALI include sepsis, mechanical ventilation, massive transfusion, and a positive fluid balance (Table 15.2).

Table 15.2 Patient-related risk factors for transfusion-related acute lung injury

	Reference	Type of study	Odds ratio [CI] (when given)
Sepsis			
	[24]	Retrospective	N/A
	[13]	Prospective	N/A
	[17]	Retrospective	OR 2.5 [1.2–5.2]
Shock			
	[15]	Prospective	OR 4.2 [1.7–10.6]
Mechanical ventilation			
	[25]	Retrospective	N/A
	[17]	Retrospective	OR 3.0 [1.3–7.1]
Peak pressure >30 cm H$_2$O	[15]	Prospective	OR 5.6 [2.1–14.9]
Cardiac surgery			
Emergency	[17]	Retrospective	OR 17.6 [1.8–168.5]
Elective	[15]	Prospective	OR 3.3 [1.21–9.2]
Time on bypass	[26]	Prospective	OR 1.0 [1.0–1.03]
Hematologic malignancy			
	[24]	Retrospective	N/A
	[17]	Retrospective	OR 13.1 [2.7–63.8]
	[27]	Retrospective	N/A
Massive transfusion			
	[17]	Retrospective	OR 4.5 [2.1–9.8]
Positive fluid balance			
	[15]	Prospective case	OR 1.17 [1.08–1.28] (increment per L)
Liver failure			
	[22]	Retrospective	OR 13.1 [2.7–63.8]
Liver transplant surgery	[15]	Prospective	OR 6.7 [1.3–35.7]

N/A not available

Patients on mechanical ventilation seem particularly prone to develop lung injury after transfusion of a blood product [25, 28]. In experimental TRALI, mechanical ventilation synergistically augmented lung injury, which was enhanced by the use of injurious ventilator settings [16]. In line with this, it was found that high-peak airway pressures (>30 cm H$_2$O) contribute to an increased TRALI risk [15]. Together, injurious mechanical ventilation seems to aggravate the course of a TRALI reaction.

In addition to pulmonary hits, systemic inflammatory conditions are often present in critically ill patients. Sepsis has been identified as a risk factor for TRALI in several studies in ICU patients [13, 17]. Also, the presence of shock prior to transfusion increases TRALI risk [15]. Coronary artery bypass grafting increased risk for TRALI about eight- to tenfold compared to the general patient population [17, 27]. This may be due to use of cardiopulmonary bypass [18].

There are also distinct differences between risk factors for TRALI and ALI due to other causes. There are risk factors for TRALI which are not commonly associated with ALI, such as hematologic malignancy and liver disease [22]. It is not known why these conditions strongly predisposes to TRALI, other than that these patients often receive plasma-rich products. Vice versa, well-known ALI risk factors such as pancreatitis or pneumonia were not identified as risk factors for TRALI, suggesting that TRALI is part of the ALI spectrum, but also has distinct entities.

15.3.2 Mitigating Risk of TRALI by Taking an Individualized Patient Approach

Appropriate management of critically ill patients has decreased risk of ALI. The same may hold for TRALI. The recent identification of TRALI risk factors enables ICU physicians to take an individualized approach toward their patients in need of a transfusion. Patient-focused strategies which may decrease the risk of TRALI include maintaining a restrictive fluid balance. A benefit of fluid restriction has also been shown in ALI patients and indeed suggests that fluid overload may play a role in TRALI pathogenesis [29]. However, shock prior to transfusion should also be avoided when possible. Decreasing airway pressures and maintaining low tidal volume ventilation in patients on mechanical ventilation prior to transfusion are a sensible approach, although not proven to be effective in mitigating TRALI risk in clinical trials.

15.3.3 Blood Product-Related Risk Factors for TRALI

The presence of donor anti-leukocyte antibodies in the transfused product is implicated in TRALI. Involved antibodies are mainly directed against HLA class I, HLA class II, or HNA. In a study in patients on general hospital wards, blood product-related risk factors were the transfused volume of high-titer cognate HLA class II antibody and the volume of high-titer HNA antibody [15].

Whether storage of blood products increases risk of TRALI is not clear. Bioactive lipids which increase during storage of red blood cells and platelet concentrates were shown to induce TRALI in animal models [5, 6]. A retrospective clinical study of ten TRALI patients linked the occurrence of TRALI with transfusion of blood products containing bioactive lipids [30]. However, this finding was not confirmed in other studies [15, 18]. Besides shedding of bioactive substances, red blood cells undergo changes in morphology and function during storage, including decreased chemokine scavenging and increased adhesion to the endothelium, which thereby may promote microvascular pathology in the lung [4]. However, these data are limited to preclinical TRALI models.

15.3.4 Mitigating Risk of TRALI by Modifying Blood Products

Pregnancy is the most important cause of sensitization in the donor population and 10–40 % of previously pregnant women have HLA antibodies [31]. A predominantly male donor strategy for preparation of fresh frozen plasma resulted in a reduction, but not abrogation, of TRALI cases [32, 33]. Of note, as long as a male-only donor policy is only implemented for plasma products, antibody-mediated TRALI due to red blood cell transfusion and pooled platelets are not prevented.

Whether the use of "fresh blood" reduces the risk of adverse outcome of transfusion is under debate. Although an association between transfusion of stored blood and mortality in various patient populations has been shown [34], current data on the association of stored blood and TRALI do not point toward a benefit of fresh blood [20]. Results of a clinical trial investigating the effect of fresh compared to stored red blood cells on outcome in the critically ill are expected in 2014.

15.4   Diagnosing Transfusion-Related Acute Lung Injury

All critically ill patients developing respiratory deterioration during the first 6 h after blood transfusion should be screened for the onset of TRALI. From a practical perspective, one should start to determine whether the PaO_2/FiO_2 ratio is below 300. The PaO_2 is expressed in mmHg and the FiO_2 is expressed as fraction oxygen

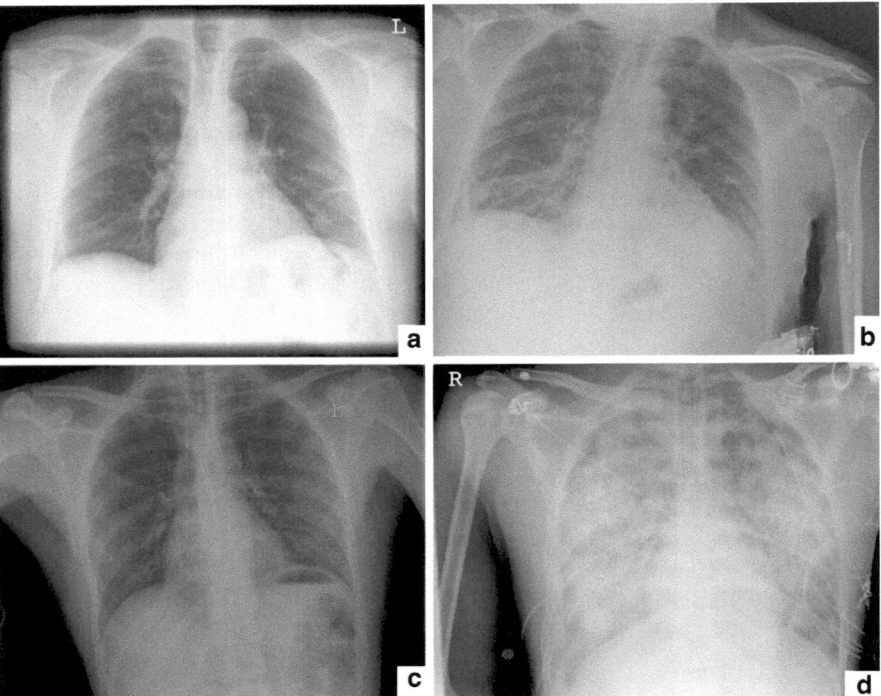

Fig. 15.1 Chest X-rays of two cases before and after onset of TRALI. Pre-onset chest X-rays (**a, c**) show normal pulmonary vasculature with no signs of pulmonary edema. Post-onset chest X-rays (**b, d**) show infiltrative changes suggestive for pulmonary edema. X-ray **b** shows subtle bilateral infiltrates while X-ray **d** shows the classical bilateral whiteout. Both cases fulfilled the definition criteria of TRALI

inspired. For example, a patient with an arterial oxygen tension of 60 mmHg and a FiO_2 of 50 % has a PaO_2/FiO_2 ratio of 120. When there is a PaO_2/FiO_2 ratio below 300, one should perform an X-ray. Although the classical "whiteout" appearance on the chest X-ray cannot be overlooked, this is not always present in TRALI (Fig. 15.1). Subtle bilateral infiltrates on the chest X-ray may be missed [35]. When the patient has bilateral infiltrates on the chest X-ray and has a PaO_2/FiO_2 ratio below 300, one should exclude hydrostatic edema [24, 36]. Differentiating between cardiogenic edema and permeability edema is not straightforward. The chest X-ray does not differentiate between these two causes. In the TRALI definition, an elevated pulmonary artery occlusion pressure of more than 18 mmHg is used to exclude hydrostatic edema. However, the use of the pulmonary artery catheter has declined. In the absence of a pulmonary artery catheter, other clinical parameters to assess the probability of the presence or absence of hydrostatic edema include central venous pressure, echocardiography, response to diuretics, and fluid balance. However, no clear guidelines exist.

Besides respiratory deterioration which is the clinical hallmark of TRALI, other symptoms may also suggest the diagnosis of TRALI, including transient neutropenia and fever [37]. Both hypotension and hypertension have been described in the onset of TRALI [38].

Diagnosing TRALI is a challenge, as illustrated by the underdiagnosing of TRALI especially when a risk factor for ALI is present [9].

15.5 Management of Suspected Transfusion-Related Acute Lung Injury

There is no specific therapy at this moment. Management of TRALI is supportive. Restrictive tidal volume ventilation and maintaining a restrictive fluid balance should be applied to avoid worsening of lung injury. In that respect, diuretics have a place in the management of TRALI.

Although treatment with steroids is anecdotally mentioned in case reports, steroids did not reduce lung injury in a mouse model of antibody-mediated TRALI [39], and clinical evidence for the therapeutic rationale of steroids in TRALI is lacking. Thereby, steroids are not recommended. Platelet activation plays a key role in TRALI pathophysiology. Acetylsalicylic acid (ASA) was found to improve outcome in an animal model of TRALI and may reduce risk of ALI [40]. However, ASA did not modify the risk of TRALI in a post hoc analysis of a cohort of critically ill patients [41]. At this moment, there is insufficient evidence to support prevention or treatment of TRALI with ASA.

The occurrence of TRALI is not a contraindication for future transfusions. Although transfusions will not improve and may in fact worsen the pulmonary condition of a TRALI patient [42, 43], it may also be necessary to continue transfusion, e.g., in the case of bleeding. When TRALI is suspected, this should be reported to the blood bank, who will start up immunologic testing in order to identify and exclude involved donors to prevent future TRALI reactions.

References

1. Goldman M, Webert KE, Arnold DM, et al. Proceedings of a consensus conference: towards an understanding of TRALI. Transfus Med Rev. 2005;19:2–31.
2. Kleinman S, Caulfield T, Chan P, et al. Toward an understanding of transfusion-related acute lung injury: statement of a consensus panel. Transfusion. 2004;44:1774–89.
3. Silliman CC. The two-event model of transfusion-related acute lung injury. Crit Care Med. 2006;34:S124–31.
4. Mangalmurti NS, Xiong Z, Hulver M, et al. Loss of red cell chemokine scavenging promotes transfusion-related lung inflammation. Blood. 2009;113:1158–66.
5. Silliman CC, Voelkel NF, Allard JD, et al. Plasma and lipids from stored packed red blood cells cause acute lung injury in an animal model. J Clin Invest. 1998;101:1458–67.
6. Silliman CC, Bjornsen AJ, Wyman TH, et al. Plasma and lipids from stored platelets cause acute lung injury in an animal model. Transfusion. 2003;43:633–40.
7. Vlaar AP, Hofstra JJ, Levi M, et al. Supernatant of aged erythrocytes causes lung inflammation and Coagulopathy in a "two-hit" in vivo syngeneic transfusion model. Anesthesiology. 2010;113:92–103.
8. Vlaar AP, Hofstra JJ, Kulik W, et al. Supernatant of stored platelets causes lung inflammation and coagulopathy in a novel in vivo transfusion model. Blood. 2010;116:1360–8.
9. Kopko PM, Marshall CS, MacKenzie MR, Holland PV, Popovsky MA. Transfusion-related acute lung injury: report of a clinical look-back investigation. JAMA. 2002;287:1968–71.
10. Engelfriet CP, Reesink HW, Brand A, et al. Transfusion-related acute lung injury (TRALI). Vox Sang. 2001;81:269–83.
11. Toy P, Popovsky MA, Abraham E, et al. Transfusion-related acute lung injury: definition and review. Crit Care Med. 2005;33:721–6.
12. Bux J, Sachs UJ. The pathogenesis of transfusion-related acute lung injury (TRALI). Br J Haematol. 2007;136:788–99.
13. Gajic O, Rana R, Winters JL, et al. Transfusion-related acute lung injury in the critically ill: prospective nested case-control study. Am J Respir Crit Care Med. 2007;176:886–91.
14. Kelher MR, Masuno T, Moore EE, et al. Plasma from stored packed red blood cells and MHC class I antibodies causes acute lung injury in a 2-event in vivo rat model. Blood. 2009;113:2079–87.
15. Toy P, Gajic O, Bacchetti P, et al. Transfusion related acute lung injury: incidence and risk factors. Blood. 2012;119:1757–67.
16. Vlaar AP, Wolthuis EK, Hofstra JJ, Roelofs JJ, Boon L, Schultz MJ, Lutter R, Juffermans NP. Mechanical ventilation aggravates transfusion-related acute lung injury induced by MHC-I class antibodies. Intensive Care Med. 2010;36:879–87.
17. Vlaar AP, Binnekade JM, Prins D, et al. Risk factors and outcome of transfusion-related acute lung injury in the critically ill: a nested case-control study. Crit Care Med. 2010;38:771–8.
18. Vlaar AP, Hofstra JJ, Determann RM, et al. The incidence, risk factors, and outcome of transfusion-related acute lung injury in a cohort of cardiac surgery patients: a prospective nested case-control study. Blood. 2011;117:4218–25.
19. Vlaar AP, Kuipers MT, Hofstra JJ, et al. Mechanical ventilation and the titer of antibodies as risk factors for the development of transfusion-related lung injury. Crit Care Res Pract. 2012;2012:720950.
20. Vlaar AP, Juffermans NP. Transfusion-related acute lung injury: a clinical review. Lancet. 2013;382:984–94.
21. Corwin HL, Gettinger A, Pearl RG, et al. The CRIT Study: anemia and blood transfusion in the critically ill–current clinical practice in the United States. Crit Care Med. 2004;32:39–52.
22. Benson AB, Austin GL, Berg M, et al. Transfusion-related acute lung injury in ICU patients admitted with gastrointestinal bleeding. Intensive Care Med. 2010;36:1710–7.
23. Henderson RA, Pinder L. Acute transfusion reactions. N Z Med J. 1990;103:509–11.
24. Rana R, Fernandez-Perez ER, Khan SA, et al. Transfusion-related acute lung injury and pulmonary edema in critically ill patients: a retrospective study. Transfusion. 2006;46:1478–83.

25. Gajic O, Rana R, Mendez JL, et al. Acute lung injury after blood transfusion in mechanically ventilated patients. Transfusion. 2004;44:1468–74.
26. Vlaar AP, Hofstra JJ, Determann RM, et al. Transfusion-related acute lung injury in cardiac surgery patients is characterized by pulmonary inflammation and coagulopathy: a prospective nested case-control study. Crit Care Med. 2012;40:2813–20.
27. Silliman CC, Boshkov LK, Mehdizadehkashi Z, et al. Transfusion-related acute lung injury: epidemiology and a prospective analysis of etiologic factors. Blood. 2003;101:454–62.
28. Dara SI, Rana R, Afessa B, Moore SB, Gajic O. Fresh frozen plasma transfusion in critically ill medical patients with coagulopathy. Crit Care Med. 2005;33:2667–71.
29. Sakr Y, Vincent JL, Reinhart K, et al. High tidal volume and positive fluid balance are associated with worse outcome in acute lung injury. Chest. 2005;128:3098–108.
30. Silliman CC, Paterson AJ, Dickey WO, et al. The association of biologically active lipids with the development of transfusion-related acute lung injury: a retrospective study. Transfusion. 1997;37:719–26.
31. Triulzi DJ, Kleinman S, Kakaiya RM, et al. The effect of previous pregnancy and transfusion on HLA alloimmunization in blood donors: implications for a transfusion-related acute lung injury risk reduction strategy. Transfusion. 2009;49:1825–35.
32. Eder AF, Herron Jr RM, Strupp A, et al. Effective reduction of transfusion-related acute lung injury risk with male-predominant plasma strategy in the American Red Cross (2006–2008). Transfusion. 2010;50:1732–42.
33. Wright SE, Snowden CP, Athey SC, et al. Acute lung injury after ruptured abdominal aortic aneurysm repair: the effect of excluding donations from females from the production of fresh frozen plasma. Crit Care Med. 2008;36:1796–802.
34. Wang D, Sun J, Solomon SB, Klein HG, Natanson C. Transfusion of older stored blood and risk of death: a meta-analysis. Transfusion. 2012;52:1184–95.
35. Vlaar AP, Porcelijn L, Van Rooijen SI, Lardy NM, Kersten MJ, Juffermans NP. The divergent clinical presentations of transfusion-related acute lung injury illustrated by two case reports. Med Sci Monit. 2010;16:CS129–34.
36. Li G, Rachmale S, Kojicic M, et al. Incidence and transfusion risk factors for transfusion-associated circulatory overload among medical intensive care unit patients. Transfusion. 2011;51:338–43.
37. Nakagawa M, Toy P. Acute and transient decrease in neutrophil count in transfusion-related acute lung injury: cases at one hospital. Transfusion. 2004;44:1689–94.
38. Moore SB. Transfusion-related acute lung injury (TRALI): clinical presentation, treatment, and prognosis. Crit Care Med. 2006;34:S114–7.
39. Muller MC, Tuinman PR, van der Sluijs KF, et al. Methylprednisolone fails to attenuate lung injury in a mouse model of transfusion related acute lung injury. Transfusion. 2014;54:996–1001.
40. Looney MR, Nguyen JX, Hu Y, et al. Platelet depletion and aspirin treatment protect mice in a two-event model of transfusion-related acute lung injury. J Clin Invest. 2009;119:3450–61.
41. Tuinman PR, Vlaar AP, Binnenkade JM, Juffermans NP. The effect of aspirin in transfusion-related acute lung injury in critically ill patients. Anaesthesia. 2012;67:594–9.
42. Gong MN, Thompson BT, Williams P, et al. Clinical predictors of and mortality in acute respiratory distress syndrome: potential role of red cell transfusion. Crit Care Med. 2005;33:1191–8.
43. Silverboard H, Aisiku I, Martin GS, et al. The role of acute blood transfusion in the development of acute respiratory distress syndrome in patients with severe trauma. J Trauma. 2005; 59:717–23.

Leanne Clifford and Daryl J. Kor

Abstract

Transfusion-associated circulatory overload (TACO) remains a leading cause of transfusion-related morbidity and mortality, accounting for 21 % of the transfusion-related fatalities reported to the United States Federal Drug Administration in 2012. While its constellation of symptoms has been recognized for over half a century, effective preventative and/or therapeutic interventions for patients with or at risk for TACO remain limited. Presently, we are primarily left with supportive cares such as oxygen supplementation and ventilator support when needed. The intensive care unit (ICU) remains one of the highest utilizers of blood products in the hospital, with one out of every two patients receiving at least one allogeneic blood component during their ICU admission. As such, critical care physicians are in a privileged position whereby accurate identification of TACO cases may not only improve patient outcomes, but may also contribute meaningfully to our understanding of TACO's epidemiology, pathophysiology, and true attributable burden. Improved case recognition will ultimately depend upon the development and acceptance of a consensus definition for TACO. In the absence of any proven therapeutic measures for TACO, perhaps the most appropriate preventative strategy is the avoidance of unnecessary transfusions through the use of conservative, evidence-based transfusion practices.

L. Clifford, BM, MSc • D.J. Kor, MD (✉)
Department of Anesthesiology, Mayo Clinic,
Rochester, 200 First St SW, Rochester, MN 55905, USA
e-mail: kor.daryl@mayo.edu

© Springer International Publishing Switzerland 2015
N.P. Juffermans, T.S. Walsh (eds.), *Transfusion in the Intensive Care Unit*,
DOI 10.1007/978-3-319-08735-1_16

16.1   Background

Physicians have been transfusing critically ill patients for generations. While transfusion practice has been refined over recent years [1, 2], the intensive care unit (ICU) environment remains one of the highest utilizers of blood products in the hospital [3]. In the United States, an estimated 24,000,000 blood products are transfused each year [4] with approximately 40 % of critically ill patients receiving at least one unit of red blood cells (RBC) [5] and one out of every two patients receiving at least one allogeneic blood product during their ICU admission [6]. Increasingly, however, the risk-to-benefit ratio of blood product administration is debated, particularly in the context of RBC transfusion for stable anemia [7]. Fortunately, due to advances in donor screening, blood product testing, treatment and storage techniques, and transfusion medicine practices, transfusion today is safer than ever, particularly with regard to the vertical transmission of infectious disease [4, 8].

Consequent to these trends, transfusion-associated circulatory overload (TACO) – a clinical syndrome characterized by pulmonary edema and hypoxemic respiratory insufficiency – has gained increasing attention as one the more serious complications of transfusion therapies. Indeed in 2012, the United States Food and Drug Administration (FDA) identified TACO as the second leading cause of transfusion-related death, accounting for 21 % of reported fatalities [4]. Meanwhile, in the United Kingdom, the Serious Hazards of Transfusion (SHOT) annual report noted TACO to be the leading cause of fatalities, accounting for an astonishing 67 % [8]. Though its recognition as an important transfusion-related complication has improved, the epidemiology, mechanisms, and attributable burden of TACO remain poorly defined and incompletely understood [9, 10]. In this chapter, we provide a contemporary review of the epidemiology of TACO with specific emphasis on its prevalence, risk factors, management, and outcomes.

16.2   TACO: Definition and Diagnosis

The absence of a uniform definition for TACO has been a major obstacle to achieving a consistent and reliable diagnosis in clinical practice, as well as to the conduct of TACO-related research. Historically, TACO has been broadly characterized by acute respiratory distress, tachycardia, and hypertension following blood product administration [2]. Though a seemingly straightforward constellation of symptoms, it is a common misconception that TACO is an easy diagnosis to make. To the contrary, multiple lines of evidence suggest that TACO diagnoses are frequently either missed entirely or misdiagnosed (e.g., transfusion-related acute lung injury (TRALI) or congestive heart failure) [8, 11, 12]. In the absence of a validated consensus definition, the most widely accepted criteria for TACO are those published in 2010 by the National Healthcare Safety Network (Table 16.1) [13]. Specifically, patients are required to have new onset or exacerbation of at least three of the following six criteria during or within 6 h of completing a transfusion episode:

Table 16.1 Transfusion-associated circulatory overload (TACO) from the CDC National Healthcare Safety Network Biovigilance Component 2013

New onset or exacerbation of three or more of the following within 6 h of cessation of transfusion:
Acute respiratory distress (dyspnea, orthopnea, cough)
Elevated brain natriuretic peptide (BNP)
Elevated central venous pressure (CVP)
Evidence of left heart failure
Evidence of positive fluid balance
Radiographic evidence of pulmonary edema

Adapted from CDC NHSN Biovigilance Component 2013 [13]
Abbreviation: *CDC* centers for disease control

- Acute respiratory distress
- Elevated brain natriuretic peptide
- Elevated central venous pressure
- Evidence of left heart failure
- Evidence of positive fluid balance
- Radiographic evidence of pulmonary edema

In clinical practice, the application of these criteria to make a diagnosis of TACO can be challenging, particularly in the ICU setting where patients frequently have numerous cardiopulmonary comorbidities, often have significantly positive fluid balance, and may be receiving ventilatory support prior to the onset of transfusion [1]. This difficulty is further accentuated by the similar clinical phenotype of alternate diagnoses such as TRALI and the acute respiratory distress syndrome (ARDS) which also manifest with pulmonary edema and hypoxemia. Though no pathognomonic findings for the diagnosis of TACO exist, various clinical signs and parameters, when considered collectively, may support the identification of TACO cases and help differentiate them from TRALI and ARDS (Table 16.2) [14].

In an effort to further address the challenges associated with making a diagnosis of TACO, various authors have attempted to develop tools and/or streamlined clinical practice guidelines to facilitate case identification. In a 2012 single-center cohort study, Andrzejewski and colleagues evaluated how trends in vital sign measurements may be used as clinical prompts to herald the onset of TACO [15]. When categorized into easy-to-apply clinical cutoffs, the investigators identified (1) an increase in systolic blood pressure ≥ 15 mmHg, (2) an increase in pulse pressure (PP) ≥ 8 mmHg, or (3) end-of-transfusion PP measurement ≥ 65 mmHg, as occurring with significantly greater frequency in patients who went on to develop TACO [15].

In addition, these authors also examined the absolute values, as well as changes in NT-pro-brain natriuretic peptide (NT-proBNP) in patients with TACO compared to transfused controls without respiratory insufficiency [15]. They identified patients with TACO as having significantly higher levels of NT-proBNP in the immediate and delayed posttransfusion period (11.5 ± 29.6 pg/mL vs. 3.0 ± 2.8 pg/mL, $p = 0.012$, and 14.8 ± 37.5 pg/mL vs. 5.0 ± 4.8 pg/mL; $p = 0.025$). TACO patients also demonstrated a higher ratio of NT-proBNP immediately after transfusion and at a more delayed

Table 16.2 Clinical features facilitating the differentiation of TACO and TRALI

Feature	TACO	TRALI
Echocardiography	EF < 40 %, E/e' > 15	EF > 40 %, E/e' ≤ 15
PCWP	>18 mmHg	≤18 mmHg
Neck veins	Distended	Normal
Chest exam	Rales, S3	Rales, No S3
Chest radiograph	VPW ≥ 65 mm, CTR ≥ 0.55	VPW < 65 mm, CTR < 0.55
Fluid balance	Positive	Neutral
BNP	>1,200 pg/ml	<250 pg/ml
NT-proBNP	>3,000 pg/ml	<1,000 pg/ml
Diuretic response	Significant improvement	Inconsistent
Blood pressure	Hypertension	Hypotension
WBC	Unchanged	Transient leukopenia

Adapted from: Goldberg and Kor [14]
Abbreviations: *TACO* transfusion-associated circulatory overload, *TRALI* transfusion-related acute lung injury, *EF* ejection fraction, *E/e'* ratio of early diastolic mitral inflow velocity to early diastolic mitral annulus velocity, *PCWP* pulmonary capillary wedge pressure, *VPW* vascular pedicle width, *CTR* cardiothoracic ratio, *BNP* brain natriuretic peptide, *NT-proBNP* N-terminal pro-brain natriuretic peptide, *WBC* white blood cell count

time point (when compared to baseline) (2.6 ± 5.1 vs. 1.0 ± 0.3 and 3.8 ± 6.5 vs. 1.6 ± 1.4; $p = 0.008$ and 0.017, respectively) [15]. The potential utility of BNP has also been previously described by Zhou and colleagues, who noted that a >50 % increase in BNP levels following transfusion had a sensitivity and specificity of 81 and 89 %, respectively, for making a diagnosis of TACO versus no transfusion reaction [16]. A subsequent case-control investigation found the accuracy of posttransfusion NT-proBNP for making a diagnosis of TACO to be 87.5 % [17]. While these data support the potential utility of BNP and NT-proBNP in facilitating a diagnosis of TACO, Li and colleagues concluded that BNP and NT-proBNP have limited diagnostic value when attempting to make the more difficult distinction of TACO versus TRALI [18]. In light of these conflicting results, the role of physiologic and laboratory derangements such as those described will require additional prospective validation prior to endorsement as reliable intermediate markers of TACO.

Recognizing the existence of poor syndrome recognition, as well as the potential for leveraging a robust electronic health record (EHR) infrastructure, the authors of this chapter sought to develop an electronic screening algorithm that could facilitate the identification of TACO diagnoses [12]. In this study, a parsimonious algorithm including measures of oxygenation and respiratory distress as well as the acquisition of a chest imaging study within 12 h of a transfusion episode effectively differentiated TACO cases from complication-free transfused controls. This initial algorithm was subsequently refined through the addition of natural language processing for the chest radiograph (CXR) reports [19]. In brief, the presence of a CXR consistent with TACO – in combination with a partial pressure of arterial oxygen (PaO_2) to fraction of inspired oxygen (FiO_2) ratio (P:F ratio) of ≤292 mmHg or, in the absence of a P:F ratio, a PaO_2 ≤ 130 mmHg, oxygen saturation ≤ 96 %, or respiratory rate ≥17/

min – was found to identify cases of TACO with 100 % sensitivity and 94 % specificity in a derivation cohort [19]. While a promising approach to identifying TACO episodes, limitations include the requirement for a robust EHR and the availability of radiograph reports with informatics expertise in the domain of natural language processing. Moreover, the external validity and reliability of these techniques remain untested and require further study.

16.3   Epidemiology and Burden of Disease

Historically, reported incidence rates for TACO have been based upon passive reporting. Reliance on these mechanisms suggested that TACO is a relatively rare event (incidence <1 %) [20]. However, in 2005 blood centers began reporting TACO to the FDA as a specific cause of transfusion-related death [4]. Since this time, TACO has received increased recognition as an important cause of transfusion-related morbidity and mortality. Indeed, more contemporary investigations utilizing active surveillance have suggested TACO incidence rates ranging from 4 to 8 % [11, 21]. As an example, in a single-center, 1-month prospective cohort study evaluating patients transfused with plasma outside of the operating room and emergency department environments, Narick and colleagues identified a TACO incidence rate of 4.8 % [11]. Of concern, none of the cases identified by the investigating authors had been reported to the hospital blood bank by the responsible clinical team. Similarly, using highly sensitive TACO screening algorithms followed by manual review of all screen-positive cases, the authors of this chapter recently identified a TACO incidence rate of 4.3 % following intraoperative blood product administration (unpublished results). Again, none of the confirmed cases had been reported by the clinical service. Importantly, similar temporal trends are noted when evaluating the impact of TACO on patient-important outcomes. While initially accounting for as little as 2 % of all transfusion-related fatalities reported to the FDA, data from 2012 puts this figure at 21 % [4]. This makes TACO the second leading cause of transfusion-related fatalities, trailing only TRALI. Similarly, the 2012 SHOT report from the UK found TACO to be the leading cause of transfusion-associated deaths, accounting for six out of the nine (67 %) reported fatalities that year [22].

Regarding the incidence of TACO in critically ill populations, there again remains significant uncertainty. In 2011, Li and colleagues reported that 51 of 901 (6 %) patients transfused in a tertiary ICU setting developed TACO [23]. In comparison, other publications have reported incidence rates up to 11 % [24]. The difficulty in identifying cases of TACO is likely one reason why there have been such discrepancies in reported incidence rates. Bearing this in mind, the true incidence of TACO is likely best represented by the upper limits of the reported range. Together with our heightened awareness of TACO, refined diagnostic criteria as well as improved case ascertainment strategies will likely play an important role in improving our future understanding of the true epidemiology of this syndrome. Of note, a consistent finding is that TACO appears to be more common in patients who are transfused in the ICU setting as compared to the general hospital ward

[11, 25]. This may in part be explained by the higher prevalence of comorbid conditions that are thought to be risk factors for TACO, such as advanced age as well as cardiovascular and renal disease. In addition, ICU populations frequently require large-volume resuscitation and high transfusion rates, both known risk factors for TACO [23].

16.4　Pathophysiology and Risk Factors for TACO

Since its earliest reports more than 70 years ago [10], TACO's clinical manifestations of dyspnea, hypoxia, and hypertension have been suggested to result from hydrostatic pulmonary edema [10, 26]. Simply stated, transfusing too large a volume of blood at too fast an infusion rate has been postulated to result in hypervolemia, elevated left atrial pressures, alveolar flooding, and respiratory distress [23]. While this mechanism holds clear biologic plausibility, it is of interest to note that a growing number of investigations suggest the potential for TACO development in patients receiving low-volume transfusion. In 1996, Popovsky and colleagues noted that the orthopedic surgical patients who developed TACO frequently received only one or two units of RBCs [21]. Since this observation, several other authors have similarly noted that TACO can occur in the setting of low-volume or even single-unit blood-product transfusion [8, 27, 28]. While it has been postulated that such patients are simply more susceptible to circulatory overload due to pre-existing cardiac dysfunction [23], additional potentially synergistic mechanisms have been proposed as well [23].

In 2005, Singel et al. hypothesized that impaired nitric oxide (NO) metabolism in stored RBCs may lead to posttransfusion microcirculatory NO trapping [29]. Consequently, increases in vascular resistance may precipitate left ventricular dysfunction, ultimately resulting in hydrostatic pulmonary edema (TACO). These findings have been corroborated by a growing number of investigations and may partly explain the relationship between TACO and the characteristic acute hypertensive response [15, 30]. More recently, as has been described in the congestive heart failure literature [31], inflammatory mediators have been implicated in the pathogenesis of TACO [32]. This notion gained reverence in 2010 when Blumberg et al. noted a dramatic 49 % reduction in the incidence of TACO following the introduction of universal prestorage leukoreduction of RBCs [33]. It was postulated that this effect was the result of an attenuated accumulation of leukocyte- and platelet-derived inflammatory mediators due to the leukoreduction procedures. These results are perhaps further supported by the findings of Andrzejewski et al. who noted the frequent occurrence of fever in those who developed TACO [15, 32]. While interesting and hypothesis generating, the results of studies such as these will clearly require further validation. Indeed, the exact mechanism or mechanisms underlying TACO remain an area of ongoing investigation. To this point, the National Institutes of Health is currently supporting studies investigating the roles of biological and inflammatory mediators, microparticles, and free hemoglobin on pulmonary inflammation and vascular dysfunction.

Though the precise mechanisms underlying TACO remain under investigation, a number of risk factors for its development have been described. Some of the earliest reported recipient risk factors, including extremes of age (<3 or >60 year), severe chronic anemia, and plasma transfusion for the reversal of oral anticoagulant therapy, are still broadly considered predisposing characteristics for TACO [23, 26]. Chronic anemia and hemorrhagic shock are believed to be risk factors for TACO due to an associated hyperdynamic state and the relative intolerance of the cardiovascular system to acute increases in circulating blood volume. Plasma transfusion for the reversal of oral anticoagulant therapy is presumed related to TACO due to the large volume of plasma required to achieve the desired end points (frequently greater than 1–2 L). More recently, Murphy et al. associated chronic renal failure, heart failure, and transfusion in a setting of hemorrhagic shock with risk for TACO [25]. Additionally the number of blood products administered and a positive fluid balance were associated with increased rates of TACO as well [25]. Importantly, while the extremes of age appear to be at heightened risk, data from the Quebec Hemo-vigilance study highlight the fact that TACO can occur in all age groups [28]. Specifically, this investigation noted that 9 % of TACO cases occurred in transfusion recipients who were <50 years of age, 15 % in those <60 year, and approximately 7 % occurred in those aged 18–49 years [28].

16.5 Management

If TACO is suspected, the transfusion should be discontinued immediately and the institutional transfusion medicine service and/or blood bank contacted in order to initiate an appropriate workup [32, 34, 35]. This should include reserving any remaining portion of the blood product for possible laboratory testing. Treatment of the transfusion recipient remains supportive as there are no known effective therapeutic interventions for established TACO. Therefore, current treatments are geared toward managing these events as you would a patient with acute decompensated heart failure, including oxygen supplementation, ventilator support when needed, and, as hemodynamic status will allow, measures to achieve a negative fluid balance [36]. In light of the fact that most patients with TACO present with hypertension, the use of intravenous diuretics to enhance urine output and foster negative fluid balance is generally recommended. Noninvasive ventilation with continuous positive airway pressure has been shown to reduce the need for endotracheal intubation as well as mortality in patients with acute hypoxemic respiratory insufficiency resulting from congestive heart failure [37, 38]. As such, we would recommend the consideration of noninvasive ventilatory strategies in TACO cases as well, provided the patient remains hemodynamically stable. For patients with a concomitant respiratory and/or metabolic acidosis or associated shock, more controlled ventilatory strategies should be considered [39, 40]. When invasive ventilatory support is required, lung-protective ventilation strategies should be employed using low tidal volume ventilation (≤6 ml per kg of ideal body weight) while maintaining an inspiratory plateau pressure of ≤30 cm H_2O [41, 42]. Data relating to appropriate levels of positive end expiratory pressure (PEEP) are insufficient to provide meaningful evidence-based recommendations in the setting of TACO. Although elevated PEEP levels (>5 cm H_2O) are often utilized in the setting of congestive heart failure, there is little data to suggest that this provides substantial benefit in the setting of TACO.

16.6 Outcomes

While the true attributable burden of TACO remains incompletely defined, it is generally agreed that it has a significant impact on many patient-important outcomes. To this point, Robillard and colleagues have reported that 21 % of TACO cases reported to the Quebec Hemovigilance System were classified as "life threatening" [28]. Similarly, the United Kingdom's Serious Hazards of Transfusion committee reported that 13 out of 15 TACO cases indentified in 2010 resulted in ICU admission [22]. Additional reports have further shown that TACO results in increased ICU and hospital lengths of stay. With regard to mortality, similar associations are believed to exist. In recent years, hemovigilance reports to the FDA have shown TACO to be responsible for a far greater proportion of transfusion-related deaths than was perhaps initially appreciated [4]. Specifically, for the fiscal year of 2012, 21 % of the transfusion-related fatalities reported to the US FDA were secondary to TACO [4]. This attributable mortality was second only to TRALI [4]. Notably, other national hemovigilance programs have reported similar findings. In the United Kingdom, TACO is recognized as the leading cause of transfusion-related fatalities, accounting for six of the nine reported deaths in 2011 [22]. The French experience suggested a case fatality rate of 3.6 % in 2002 [43]. In 2008, Quebec reported a TACO case fatality rate of 1.4 % [28]. This was followed by a 2011 report from the University of Pittsburgh Medical Center which reported an alarming case fatality rate of 8.3 % [11]. In further support of the impact of TACO on transfusion-recipient mortality, Murphy and colleagues recently performed a case-control study and noted that patients with TACO had a significantly increased risk of in-hospital death (Hazard ratio 3.20; 95 % CI, 1.23–8.10) [25]. In this study, TACO survivors also had longer hospital and ICU lengths of stay, even after controlling for Acute Physiology and Chronic Health Evaluation-II scores [25]. In contrast, when ICU populations were studied in a single-center observational study, Li and colleagues failed to identify a significant difference in mortality when comparing transfusion recipients with and without TACO [44]. However, the authors did identify significantly longer ICU and hospital lengths of stay in the TACO cohort [44]. While the reason for this discrepant mortality results remains unclear, the sum of available literature would certainly seem to support that TACO has a substantial impact on patient-important outcomes.

16.7 Prevention

Consideration of several critical points at or around the time of transfusion may prove essential in the prevention of consequent TACO. Most importantly, the avoidance of unnecessary transfusions through the use of conservative, evidence-based transfusion practices [6, 45] is expected to have the most meaningful impact on TACO prevention [32, 46]. While transfusion therapies can be lifesaving in the setting of acute hemorrhage, it has been estimated that 90 % of ICU RBC transfusions occur in the context of stable anemia [3, 5, 7]. Similarly, Dzik and colleagues have suggested that the majority of plasma transfusions occur in the absence of evidence-based indications [47]. This, coupled with the abundance of data demonstrating that conservative transfusion practices are associated with better short- and long-term outcomes, gives weight to the argument that in many clinical situations transfusion can be avoided all together [1, 26]. In situations whereby transfusion is truly necessary, providers should endeavor to assess the individual patients' risk for TACO and adjust clinical management accordingly. Such assessment should include careful review of the patients past medical history, specifically focusing on evidence of congestive heart failure, renal insufficiency, and fluid status. Notably, a recent investigation also suggested the need for greater vigilance by the clinical team when assessing risk for TACO [15, 32, 46, 48]. Specifically, the authors noted that most of the transfusion recipients who developed TACO had at least one underlying risk factor at the time of transfusion. Despite this risk, physicians rarely assessed their patients' fluid status before ordering a transfusion, often ordered large volumes of transfusions at excessive rates, and infrequently ordered diuretic therapy [48].

In hemodynamically stable at-risk populations, it is recommended that (1) only one unit of RBCs be transfused at a time, (2) a slower rate of transfusion be used, and (3) physicians consider administration of pre- or peri-transfusion diuretics to offset the associated increase in circulating blood volume [15, 46]. The AABB specifically recommend a rate of 150–300 m/h, with a reduced rate of 1 ml/kg/h in patients with known cardiac dysfunction [2]. While such recommendations make good physiologic sense, it must be acknowledged that there are very limited data supporting the efficacy of these interventions in terms of TACO prevention. Moreover, the application of these guidelines can occasionally be challenging, particularly in the setting of significant hemorrhage. With regard to the use of diuretics, we again stress that this has not been widely tested in a controlled manner. Indeed, the limited available data has questioned the efficacy of this practice [23]. Furthermore, in those with hypotension, electrolyte abnormalities, or cardiac arrhythmias, the potential adverse effects associated with pharmacologically assisted diuresis must be considered.

Additional TACO mitigation strategies are under evaluation as well. Examples include the use of reduced volume, concentrated blood products [49], as well as the preferential use of factor concentrates as alternatives to plasma transfusion [50]. These blood component alternatives are particularly attractive in patients who may not tolerate the volume frequently associated with plasma transfusion. Importantly, however, these strategies have also not yet undergone thorough evaluation and as such cannot yet be broadly endorsed. Finally, we would strongly advocate that all patients being transfused with blood products should undergo frequent nursing assessments both during the transfusion episode as well as in the early posttransfusion period as a method for potentially averting more severe forms of TACO through early recognition and appropriate intervention.

16.8 Enhancing Recognition and Understanding of TACO

Although interest in the epidemiology of TACO and its underlying mechanisms is increasing, substantial knowledge gaps remain. Pivotal to enhancing our recognition and understanding of TACO is the adoption of a unified definition. At this time, the definitions put forth by the Centers for Disease Control, National Healthcare Safety Network Manual on Transfusion Biovigilance [13] appear to have garnered the most support. Importantly, however, the subjective nature and lack of specific diagnostic criteria for many of the components of this definition (e.g., dyspnea, BNP, CVP, fluid balance) remain a major limitation. As such, further refinements in this definition are still needed.

16.9 Conclusion

Transfusion-associated circulatory overload remains one of the leading causes of transfusion-related morbidity and mortality [4, 22]. While its constellation of symptoms has been recognized for over half a century [10], effective preventative strategies and/or therapeutic interventions for patients with or at risk for TACO remain limited. A major barrier to the prevention and management of TACO continues to be the lack of a precise and broadly endorsed definition leading to subsequent failure to accurately identify cases in clinical practice. Thus, a key step forward in the TACO domain will be a refinement in its definition with the expectation of this resulting in improved syndrome recognition, surveillance, and pathophysiologic understanding. Effective prevention should start with conservative, evidence-based transfusion practices [2], which may prove paramount in mitigating the impact of TACO. Sustained efforts focused on improving the accuracy of TACO identification as well as enhancing our understanding of the mechanisms underlying this transfusion complication should ultimately result in improved management strategies. Until this time, supportive care with oxygen supplementation and ventilator support when indicated remains the therapeutic mainstays.

References

1. Hebert PC, et al. A multicenter, randomized, controlled clinical trial of transfusion requirements in critical care. Transfusion Requirements in Critical Care Investigators, Canadian Critical Care Trials Group. N Engl J Med. 1999;340(6):409–17.
2. Roback J, et al. AABB technical manual. 16th ed. Bethesda: American Association of Blood Banks; 2011.
3. Walsh TS, et al. Red cell requirements for intensive care units adhering to evidence-based transfusion guidelines. Transfusion. 2004;44(10):1405–11.
4. Fatalities reported to FDA following blood collection and transfusion: annual summary for fiscal year 2012. 17 July 2013. Available from: http://www.fda.gov/BiologicsBloodVaccines/SafetyAvailability/ReportaProblem/TransfusionDonationFatalities/ucm346639.htm.
5. Corwin HL, et al. The CRIT Study: anemia and blood transfusion in the critically ill–current clinical practice in the United States. Crit Care Med. 2004;32(1):39–52.

6. Napolitano LM, Kurek SL, Luchette FA, et al. Clinical practice guideline: red blood cell transfusion in adult trauma and critical care. Crit Care Med. 2009;37(12):3124–57.

7. Vincent JL, et al. Anemia and blood transfusion in critically ill patients. JAMA. 2002;288(12):1499–507.

8. Bolton-Maggs PH, Cohen H. Serious Hazards of Transfusion (SHOT) haemovigilance and progress is improving transfusion safety. Br J Haematol. 2013;163(3):303–14.

9. Popovsky MA, Taswell HF. Circulatory overload: an underdiagnosed consequence of transfusion. Transfusion. 1985;25(5):469.

10. Drummond R. Transfusion reactions and fatalities due to circulatory overloading. Br Med J. 1943;2(4314):319–22.

11. Narick C, Triulzi DJ, Yazer MH. Transfusion-associated circulatory overload after plasma transfusion. Transfusion. 2012;52(1):160–5.

12. Clifford L, et al. Electronic health record surveillance algorithms facilitate the detection of transfusion-related pulmonary complications. Transfusion. 2013;53(6):1205–16.

13. The National Healthcare Safety Network, Biovigilance Component. [cited 2013 January 3rd 2014]. 2013. Available from: http://www.cdc.gov/nhsn/PDFs/hemovigModuleProtocol_current.pdf.

14. Goldberg AD, Kor DJ. State of the art management of transfusion-related acute lung injury (TRALI). Curr Pharm Des. 2012;18(22):3273–84.

15. Andrzejewski Jr C, et al. Hemotherapy bedside biovigilance involving vital sign values and characteristics of patients with suspected transfusion reactions associated with fluid challenges: can some cases of transfusion-associated circulatory overload have proinflammatory aspects? Transfusion. 2012;52(11):2310–20.

16. Zhou L, et al. Use of B-natriuretic peptide as a diagnostic marker in the differential diagnosis of transfusion-associated circulatory overload. Transfusion. 2005;45(7):1056–63.

17. Tobian AA, et al. N-terminal pro-brain natriuretic peptide is a useful diagnostic marker for transfusion-associated circulatory overload. Transfusion. 2008;48(6):1143–50.

18. Li G, et al. The accuracy of natriuretic peptides (brain natriuretic peptide and N-terminal pro-brain natriuretic) in the differentiation between transfusion-related acute lung injury and transfusion-related circulatory overload in the critically ill. Transfusion. 2009;49(1):13–20.

19. Clifford L, et al. Natural language processing of chest radiograph reports improves the identification of transfusion-related pulmonary complications. Am J Respir Crit Care Med. 2013;187:A2218.

20. Audet A, Andrzejewski Jr C, Popovsky M. Red blood cell transfusion practices in patients undergoing orthopedic surgery: a multi-institutional analysis. Orthopedics. 1998;21(8):851–8.

21. Popovsky MA, Audet AM, Andrzejewski Jr C. Transfusion-associated circulatory overload in orthopedic surgery patients: a multi-institutional study. Immunohematology. 1996;12(2):87–9.

22. PHBBolton-Maggs (Ed), Poles D, Watt A, Thomas D, Cohen H. on behalf of the Serious Hazards of Transfusion (SHOT) Steering Group. The 2012 annual SHOT Report. 2013.

23. Li G, Rachmale S, Kojicic M. Incidence and transfusion risk factors for transfusion-associated circulatory overload among medical intensive care unit patients. Transfusion. 2011;51:338–43.

24. Rana R, et al. Transfusion related pulmonary edema in the intensive care unit. Chest. 2005;128(4):Supplement 130s.

25. Murphy EL, et al. Risk factors and outcomes in transfusion-associated circulatory overload. Am J Med. 2013;126(4):357.e29–38.

26. Vamvakas EC, Blajchman MA. Blood still kills: six strategies to further reduce allogeneic blood transfusion-related mortality. Transfus Med Rev. 2010;24(2):77–124.

27. Popovsky MA. The Emily Cooley Lecture 2009 To breathe or not to breathe-that is the question. Transfusion. 2010;50(9):2057–62.

28. Robillard P, Itaj N, Chapdelaine A. Increasing incidence of transfusion-associated circulatory overload reported to the Quebec Hemovigilance System, 2000–2006. Transfusion. 2008;48(S2):204A.

29. Singel DJ, Stamler JS. Chemical physiology of blood flow regulation by red blood cells: the role of nitric oxide and S-nitrosohemoglobin. Annu Rev Physiol. 2005;67:99–145.

30. Donadee C, et al. Nitric oxide scavenging by red blood cell microparticles and cell-free hemo-globin as a mechanism for the red cell storage lesion. Circulation. 2011;124(4):465–76.
31. Celis R, Torre-Martinez G, Torre-Amione G. Evidence for activation of immune system in heart failure: is there a role for anti-inflammatory therapy? Curr Opin Cardiol. 2008;23(3):254–60.
32. Andrzejewski C, Casey Jr MA, Popovsky MA. How we view and approach transfusion-associated circulatory overload: pathogenesis, diagnosis, management, mitigation, and prevention. Transfusion. 2013;53(12):3037–47.
33. Blumberg N, et al. An association between decreased cardiopulmonary complications (transfusion-related acute lung injury and transfusion-associated circulatory overload) and implementation of universal leukoreduction of blood transfusions. Transfusion. 2010;50(12):2738–44.
34. Popovsky M. Transfusion-associated circulatory overload. In: Popovsky M, editor. Transfusion reactions. Bethesda: AABB Press; 2012. p. 326–37.
35. AABB. Standards for blood banks and transfusion services. 28th ed. Bethesda: American Association of Blood Banks; 2012.
36. Jessup M, et al. 2009 focused update: ACCF/AHA Guidelines for the Diagnosis and Management of Heart Failure in Adults: a report of the American College of Cardiology Foundation/American Heart Association Task Force on Practice Guidelines: developed in collaboration with the International Society for Heart and Lung Transplantation. Circulation. 2009;119(14):1977–2016.
37. Winck JC, et al. Efficacy and safety of non-invasive ventilation in the treatment of acute cardiogenic pulmonary edema–a systematic review and meta-analysis. Crit Care. 2006;10(2):R69.
38. Masip J, et al. Noninvasive ventilation in acute cardiogenic pulmonary edema: systematic review and meta-analysis. JAMA. 2005;294(24):3124–30.
39. Schmickl CN, et al. The accuracy and efficiency of electronic screening for recruitment into a clinical trial on COPD. Respir Med. 2011;105(10):1501–6.
40. Peter JV, et al. Effect of non-invasive positive pressure ventilation (NIPPV) on mortality in patients with acute cardiogenic pulmonary oedema: a meta-analysis. Lancet. 2006;367(9517):1155–63.
41. Putensen C, et al. Meta-analysis: ventilation strategies and outcomes of the acute respiratory distress syndrome and acute lung injury. Ann Intern Med. 2009;151(8):566–76.
42. Ventilation with lower tidal volumes as compared with traditional tidal volumes for acute lung injury and the acute respiratory distress syndrome. The Acute Respiratory Distress Syndrome Network. N Engl J Med. 2000;342(18):1301–8.
43. David B. Haemovigilance: a comparison of three national systems. In: Proceeding of the 27th congress of the international society of blood transfusion. Vancouver; 2002.
44. Li G, et al. Long-term survival and quality of life after transfusion-associated pulmonary edema in critically ill medical patients. Chest. 2010;137(4):783–9.
45. Carson JL, et al. Red blood cell transfusion: a clinical practice guideline from the AABB*. Ann Intern Med. 2012;157(1):49–58.
46. Alam A, et al. The prevention of transfusion-associated circulatory overload. Transfus Med Rev. 2013;27(2):105–12.
47. Dzik W, Rao A. Why do physicians request fresh frozen plasma? Transfusion. 2004;44(9):1393–4.
48. Lieberman L, et al. A retrospective review of patient factors, transfusion practices, and outcomes in patients with transfusion-associated circulatory overload. Transfus Med Rev. 2013;27(4):206–12.
49. Silvergleid AJ. Up-to-date: transfusion reactions caused by chemical and physical agents. Transfusion Associated Circulatory Overload 2013. 10 Sept 2013. Available from: http://www.uptodate.com/contents/transfusion-reactions-caused-by-chemical-and-physical-agents?source=see_link&anchor=H2#H2.
50. Franchini M, Lippi G. Prothrombin complex concentrates: an update. Blood Transfus. 2010;8(3):149–54.

Index

A

Acetylsalicylic acid (ASA), 167
Acidosis, 103, 110, 111
Acute respiratory distress
    syndrome (ARDS), 173
Acute traumatic coagulopathy (ATC)
  base deficit, 104–105
  blood pressure target, 114–115
  conventional treatment, 109–110
  endothelial glycocalyx degradation, 107
  fibrinogen, 105
  fibrinolysis, 106
  fresh frozen plasma, 110–111
  haemostatic agents, 113–114
  injury severity score, 104–105
  massive transfusion protocols, 112–113
  murine model, 105
  optimal blood product ratio, 111–112
  tissue hypoperfusion, 104
  vascular endothelium, 106
Acute upper gastrointestinal
    bleeding (AUGIB)
  antifibrinolytics, 132–133
  haemorrhage protocols, 133–134
  liver cirrhosis
    AVH, 123
    coagulopathy of, 124–126
  non-variceal bleeding, 132
  plasma transfusion, 131–132
  platelet transfusions
    antiplatelet therapy, 131
    thrombocytopenia, 130–131
  rebleeding, 123
  red blood cell transfusion
    guidelines for, 128
    mechanisms of harm, 130
    observational studies, 128–129
    purpose of, 127–128
    randomised trial evidence, 129–130
  variceal bleeding, 126–127

Acute variceal haemorrhage (AVH), 122, 123
Anaphylaxis, 143
Anemia
  abnormal RBC maturation, 9
  in cardiac surgery, 36–37
  of chronic disease, 7
  in congestive heart failure, 26–27
  elderly population
    consequences, 63–64
    etiology, 61–62
    NHANES III, 59–60
    physiologic response, 62–63
    prevalence, 59–60
  ESAs, 79–81
  etiology, 6
  HBOCs
    adverse effects, 86
    cellular, 85–86
    characteristics of, 82–83
    first-generation, 82
    Hemolink, 84
    Hemopure, 83
    hemorrhagic shock, 81
    human cross-linked hemoglobin, 82
    human-derived pyridoxylated
      hemoglobin polyoxyethylene
      conjugate, 85
    human-induced pluripotent
      stem cells, 86
    MP4/Hemospan, 84–85
    Oxyglobin, 83, 87
    PolyHeme, 84
    recombinant human hemoglobin, 85
    Sanguinate, 83–84
    second-generation, 83
  hemodilution, 10
  hemorrhagic losses, 7
  incidence, 94
  increased RBC destruction, 9–10
  inflammation, 77

© Springer International Publishing Switzerland 2015
N.P. Juffermans, T.S. Walsh (eds.), *Transfusion in the Intensive Care Unit*,
DOI 10.1007/978-3-319-08735-1

Anemia (*cont.*)
  in injured brain, 46–47
  iron supplementation, 78–79
  in normal brain, 46
  and oxygen debt, 72–73
  phlebotomy losses, 7
  red cell production, 8
  red cell survival, 97
  schematic diagram, 6
  in sepsis, 15
Anemia of chronic disease (ACD), 7
Anticalin, 79
Antifibrinolytics, 132–133
Antiplatelet therapy, 131
Aphaeresis, 143
ATC. *See* Acute traumatic coagulopathy
    (ATC)
AUGIB. *See* Acute upper gastrointestinal
    bleeding (AUGIB)

B
Blood conservation devices, 97–98
Blood-sparing strategies
  arterial line systems, 97
  blood sampling, 96
  blood use optimisation, 96–97
  evidence for blood conservation devices,
    97–98
  haemodilution and haemorrhage, 95
  phlebotomy, 94–95
  restrictive transfusion practice, 94–96
  small volume blood tubes, 98
  transfusion frequency, 94
Brain injury
  anemia in
    etiology, 48
    ischemic stroke, 47–48
    physiology, 46–47
    traumatic brain injury, 48–49
  neurocritical care studies, 54–55
  oxygen transport, 46–47
  RBC transfusion
    effects, 50
    in intracranial hemorrhage, 53–54
    in ischemic stroke, 51–52
    in traumatic brain injury, 52

C
Cardiac disease
  hemoglobin transfusion
    goal of, 30
    indication, 29

    observational studies, 28
    randomized controlled trials, 28
  oxygen consumption, 26
  pathophysiology of anemia, 26–27
Cardiac surgery
  anemia, 36–37
  red blood cell transfusion
    clinical practice, 37–38
    clinical studies, 37
    observational studies, 38–39
    randomised controlled trials, 41–42
Cardiorenal anemia syndrome, 27
Cellular HBOCs, 85–86
Central venous oxygen saturation (ScvO₂)
  anemia and oxygen debt, 72–73
  factors, 73–74
  haemoglobin level, 72
  haemorrhage, 73
  isovolaemic haemodilution, 73
  oxygen imbalance, 74
  red blood cells, 74
Chronic kidney disease (CKD), 67
Congestive heart failure (CHF), 27

D
Disseminated intravascular coagulation (DIC),
    102

E
Elderly population, red blood cell transfusion
  anemia (*see* Anemia)
  clinical guidelines, 66–67
  randomized controlled trials
    cardiovascular risk factors, 64
    Kaplan-Meier estimate, 66
    liberal-strategy group, 64–65
    mortality rate, 66
    postoperative hemoglobin level, 65
    restrictive-strategy group, 64–65
Epoetin alpha therapy, 80
Erythrocyte zinc protoporphyrin (eZPP), 78
Erythropoiesis, 8
Erythropoiesis-stimulating agents (ESAs),
    79–81
Erythropoietin, 26, 81

F
Fibrinogen, 105
Fibrinolysis, 106
Fresh frozen plasma (FFP) transfusion
  ATC, 110–111

bleeding risk, 154–155
coagulopathy
    dose recommendations, 156
    evidence-based transfusion, 156–157
critical illness
    concurrent bleeding, 154
    disordered coagulation, 152
    donor leukocytes, 153
    factor concentrations, 152
    indications, 153
    international normalised ratio, 151
    plasmapheresis, 152
    reversal of warfarin anticoagulation,
        153
    single-factor deficiencies, 153
    volume expansion, 154
ICU, 1
risks, 157–158
traumatic bleeding, 2
Functional iron deficiency (FID), 78

H
Haemostatic agents, 113–114
Hemoglobin-based oxygen carriers (HBOCs)
    adverse effects, 86
    cellular, 85–86
    characteristics of, 82–83
    first-generation, 82
    Hemolink, 84
    Hemopure, 83
    hemorrhagic shock, 81
    human cross-linked hemoglobin, 82
    human-derived pyridoxylated hemoglobin
        polyoxyethylene conjugate, 85
    human-induced pluripotent stem cells, 86
    MP4/Hemospan, 84–85
    Oxyglobin, 87
    PolyHeme, 84
    recombinant human hemoglobin, 85
    Sanguinate, 83–84
    second-generation, 83
Hemolink, 84
Hemolysis, 9–10
Hemopure, 83
Hepcidin, 78–79
Human cross-linked hemoglobin
    (DCLHb), 82
Human-derived pyridoxylated hemoglobin
    polyoxyethylene conjugate, 85
Human-induced pluripotent stem (hiPS) cells,
    86
Hyperfibrinolysis, 106
Hypersplenism, 143

I
Iron supplementation, 78–79
Ischemic stroke, 48, 51–52

L
Leucodepletion, 95
Liver cirrhosis
    acute variceal haemorrhage, 123
    coagulopathy of
        haemorrhagic phenotype, 125
        rebalanced haemostasis, 124
        thrombin generation, 124
        thrombosis, 125–126
    use of blood components, 127

M
Maximum surgical blood ordering schedules
    (MSBOS), 96–97
Mild hypothermia, 103
MP4/Hemospan, 84–85

N
Near-infrared spectroscopy (NIRS), 17
Non-cardiac surgery, red cell transfusion,
    39–41
Non-variceal upper GI bleeding, 132
NT-pro-brain natriuretic peptide (NT-proBNP),
    173–174

O
Optimal blood product ratio, 111–112
Orthogonal polarization spectral (OPS)
    imaging, 17
Oxyglobin, 83, 87

P
Packed red blood cells (PRBC), 110
Perioperative and peri-procedural transfusion,
    145
Permissive hypotension, 114
Plasma transfusion, AUGIB, 131–132
Platelet aggregometry, 109
Platelet transfusions
    aphaeresis, 143
    AUGIB
        antiplatelet therapy, 131
        thrombocytopenia, 130–131
    bleeding patients, 145
    critical care patients, 140, 142

Platelet transfusions (*cont.*)
    critically ill adults, 145–146
    critically ill neonates and
            children, 146–147
    glycoprotein receptor, 139
    hypersplenism, 143
    perioperative and peri-procedural
            transfusion, 145
    platelet function, 140–141
    platelet number, 140
    primary haemostasis, 139
    procoagulant factors, 140
    prophylactic transfusion, 144
    risks of, 143–144
    thrombocytopenia, 141–142
PolyHeme, 84
Positive end expiratory pressure
        (PEEP), 177–178
Prophylactic transfusion, 130, 144, 147
Prothrombin complex concentrate
        (PCC), 113, 153

R
Recombinant human hemoglobin (rHb), 85
Red blood cell transfusion
    AUGIB
        guidelines for, 128
        mechanisms of harm, 130
        observational studies, 128–129
        purpose of, 127–128
        randomised trial evidence, 129–130
    brain injury
        effects, 50
        in intracranial hemorrhage, 53–54
        in ischemic stroke, 51–52
        in traumatic brain injury, 52
    cardiac disease
        goal of, 30
        indication, 29
        observational studies, 28
        randomized controlled trials, 28
    cardiac surgery
        clinical practice, 37–38
        clinical studies, 37
        observational studies, 38–39
        randomised controlled trials, 41–42
    elderly population
        anemia (*see* Anemia)
        clinical guidelines, 66–67
        randomized controlled trials, 64–66
    non-cardiac surgery, 39–41

sepsis
    clinical trials, 18–19
    microcirculatory effects, 17–18
    VO_2/DO_2 and tissue oxygenation,
            15–17

S
Sanguinate, 83–84
Sepsis
    anemia in, 15
    blood transfusions
        clinical trials, 18–19
        microcirculatory effects, 17–18
        VO_2/DO_2 and tissue oxygenation,
                15–17
    oxygen delivery and consumption,
            14–15
Serum protein electrophoresis, 61
Sidestream dark-field (SDF) imaging,
        17, 18
Small volume blood tubes, 98

T
TACO. *See* Transfusion-associated circulatory
        overload (TACO)
Thrombocytopenia
    chemotherapy-associated, 141
    cirrhosis and variceal bleeding, 130–131
    heparin-induced, 141
    ICU, 142
    platelet abnormalities, 141
Thrombosis, 125–126
TIC. *See* Trauma-induced coagulopathy (TIC)
TRALI. *See* Transfusion-related acute lung
        injury (TRALI)
Tranexamic acid (TXA), 132–133
Transfusion-associated circulatory overload
        (TACO)
    burden of disease, 175–176
    definition and diagnosis, 172–175
    epidemiology, 175–176
    intensive care unit, 172
    management, 177–178
    outcomes, 178
    pathophysiology, 176–177
    prevention, 178–179
    recognition, 180
    risk factors, 176–177
Transfusion indication threshold reduction
        (TITRe 2) trial, 41, 42

Transfusion-related acute lung
    injury (TRALI)
  blood product-related risk factors, 165
  definition, 162
  diagnosis, 166–167
  incidence of, 163
  individualized patient approach, 165
  management of, 167
  modification of blood products,
      165–166
  pathogenesis, 162–163
  patient-related risk factors
    lung neutrophils, 163–164
    mechanical ventilation, 164
    plasma-rich products, 165
    sepsis, 164
    "two-hit" model, 163–164
  platelet transfusion, 144
Transfusion requirements after cardiac
    surgery (TRACS) trial
  restrictive and liberal transfusion, 41
  in sepsis, 18–19
Transfusion requirements in critical care
    (TRICC), 94–95
Transfusion-transmitted bacterial
    infection (TTBI), 144

Trauma-induced coagulopathy (TIC)
  acidosis, 103
  blood products vs. prothrombin
      time ratio, 107–108
  clot strengths, 108–109
  conventional concept of, 103
  dilutional coagulopathy, 109
  disseminated intravascular
      coagulation, 102
  mild hypothermia, 103
  platelet aggregometry, 109
  protease dysfunction, 102
  prothrombin time ratio vs.
      hospital mortality, 107
  'signature' thromboelastogram, 108
Traumatic brain injury (TBI),
    48–49, 52

U
Uraemia, 125

V
Variceal bleeding, 126–127, 130–131
Venous oxygen saturation (SvO$_2$), 16

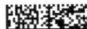